# MISO

# Cookery

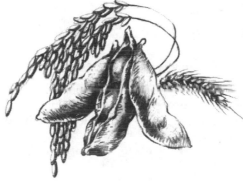

## Louise Hagler

**Book Publishing Company**
**Summertown, Tennessee**

Cover design: Warren Jefferson, Ann Hagler
Illustrations: Ann Hagler
Interior design: Louise Hagler, Michael Cook
Photos: John Guider
Food Styling: Louise Hagler, Barb Bloomfield, Michael Cook

Pictured on the front cover: Upper left picture (on top) Miso Kombu Soup, page 16, (below) North African Sweet Potato Soup, page 14

Lower right picture: Marinated Tempeh Sticks, page 64, topped with Crispy Crunchy Sweet Pepper Stir Fry, page 55

Pictured on the back cover: Corn on the Cob, page 57, Green Beans with Roasted Garlic, page 56, Mashed Potatoes, page 57, Holiday Vital Wheat Gluten Roast, page 74

Published in the United States by
Book Publishing Company
PO Box 99
Summertown, TN 38483

03 02 01 00    1 2 3 4 5 6

Hagler, Louise.
    Miso cookery / Louise Hagler.
        p.  cm.
    Includes index.
    ISBN 1-57067-102-8 (alk. paper)
        1. Cookery (Miso) 2. Vegetarian cookery. I. Title.
    TX819.M57 H34 2000
    641.6'5655--dc21                                    00-057151

Calculations for the nutritional analyses in this book are based on the average number of servings listed with the recipes and the average amount of an ingredient, if a range is called for. Calculations are rounded up to the nearest gram. If two options for an ingredient are listed, the first one is used. Not included are optional ingredients, serving suggestions, or fat used for frying, unless the amount of fat is specified in the recipe.

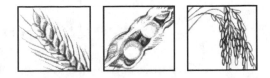

# Contents

# *Introduction*

Why miso? Miso has a rich, robust flavor, contains beneficial bacteria and enzymes, and provides high quality nutrition. It adds great taste while reducing the risk of some diseases and contributing to the creation and maintenance of a healthy body.

Miso (pronounced MEE-so) is a traditional Asian soyfood that is cultured and fermented to produce a variety of flavors, aromas, colors, and concentrations. This ancient food is rich in high-quality protein, beneficial enzymes, and friendly bacteria including lactobacillus. It comes in the form of a paste or purée, ranging from creamy beige to dark chocolate brown in color. The flavor of different varieties of miso will vary subtly in how salty, savory, rich, robust, or "meaty" they are, making them just the right complement for meatless dishes. Miso can range from sweet to savory, with full-bodied flavors like fine wines.

Unpasteurized miso is a living food containing beneficial microorganisms (probiotics) which can aid digestion and contribute to life-long health. These bacteria and their beneficial enzymes can also help the body's metabolic processes, maintain an alkaline system, help protect from cancer, and aid recovery from exposure to radiation or other pollutants, such as petroleum fumes and tobacco smoke. These beneficial components are destroyed by high heat, so pasteurized miso will contain very little of them.

A little miso goes a long way; a serving may range from a teaspoon to a tablespoon, depending on the type. If a recipe calls for a particular type of miso that you don't have on hand, try substituting one within the same color range. Each variety lends a slightly different flavor, intensity, and nutritional content. You may find you prefer one flavor or color to another after sampling a few. Sodium content will vary by manufacturer.

---

When substituting miso for salt,
you can generally use this conversion:

1 tablespoon sweet light miso = ¼ teaspoon salt

½ tablespoon dark miso = ¼ teaspoon salt

---

Lighter-colored miso, usually called sweet or mellow, is milder, less salty, and usually sweeter than darker varieties. Darker miso contains more salt, protein, and essential fatty acids, but less of the beneficial bacteria than lighter sweet or yellow miso. Traditionally, darker miso is eaten in cold months and the lighter in warm months.

The traditional process of making miso begins with cooked grains (usually rice or barley) being inoculated with *aspergillus oryzae* spores. Together, they are incubated overnight and become what is called koji (pronounced KO-jee). The next day the koji is mixed with cooked soybeans or chick-peas and salt. Soybeans add complete, high-quality protein plus all the healthful benefits of the whole soybean, while natural sea salt adds an abundance of trace minerals. This mixture is packed into wooden vats, then covered and weighted down. The fermentation process can last up to three years, if done using traditional methods.

Culturing and fermentation processes change the soybeans and rice or barley to a readily digestible form. It also transforms both bean and grain into a kind of protein booster. Since the essential amino acids in the soy and grains complement each other, the amount of protein that can be utilized by the body is increased.

Miso is salty and can be used like salt to season and enhance flavor. Since it contains a wider spectrum of flavors than just saltiness, miso can add more flavor to a dish with less sodium than salt.

The body only needs about 1,000 mg of sodium a day to replace what it normally excretes. Intake above that level can increase the chances of high blood pressure or hypertension. The amount of sodium contained in miso varies depending on the manufacturer.

| | |
|---|---|
| Table salt | 1 tsp. contains 2,000 mg sodium |
| Soy sauce | 1 tsp. contains 433 mg sodium |
| Sweet white miso | 1 tsp. contains from 147 to 290 mg sodium |
| Red miso | 1 tsp. contains from 322 to 340 mg sodium |

Miso usually contains soy protein from soybeans which, unlike animal protein, allows the regular excretion of sodium from the body, helping to keep blood pressure lower. There are recent studies suggesting that the fermentation process in miso creates antihypertensive peptides that may also help lower blood pressure.[1]

When you are buying miso, you might want to choose several different varieties in small quantities to experience the subtle differences in flavors and intensities. You will find miso in the refrigerated section of your natural food store or Asian market, usually in small plastic tubs or bags. Although traditional unpasteurized miso can be kept unrefrigerated, I would recommend keeping all types of miso refrigerated. Miso can be kept for several months to years this way.

Unpasteurized miso usually comes in plastic tubs which have a pin-prick hole in the lid to let off pressure from the fermentation. If miso comes in a sealed plastic bag, it has most likely been pasteurized. This destroys most of its beneficial bacteria and their enzymes and decreases the natural flavors and aromas. There are commercial methods of making miso that only take a few weeks, but this type of miso often contains additives and preservatives. Read the label to know what you are getting.

Miso soup is part of the traditional Japanese breakfast. Try replacing your cup of morning coffee with a cup of morning miso. Miso makes a nourishing, energizing, alkaline-producing drink to replace acid-producing, addictive coffee. While coffee gives a caffeine kick, it is followed by a let down, requiring another hit and another hit to keep you going. Miso lifts and sustains with real nourishment for the body. An alkaline blood system helps maintain good health by making it easier for the immune system to fight off disease.

There are many more special qualities attributed to this powerful food. Miso has been found to contain small amounts of vitamin $B_{12}$. A study in Japan in 1972 found that an alkaloid in miso bonds to heavy metals in the body and carries them out. There are personal accounts from people recovering from radiation treatments who suffered few ill aftereffects from the treatments while consuming miso on a regular basis during the process. There are reports from Japan that after the atomic bombs were dropped, regular miso soup drinkers did not suffer as much from the effects of radiation and recovered more quickly.[2]

More recently, miso has been shown to be useful in protecting against mammary cancer and has a potent antitumor effect, especially when used in combination with the drug tamoxifen.[3]

Studies have shown that the levels of isoflavones in fermented soybean products, such as miso, are higher than those in unfermented soy products, such as soymilk and tofu.[4]

Miso is not just for soup. It can add rich flavor to sauces, marinades, dressings, stews, roasts, and more. In order to provide all its healthful bacteria to the body, miso must not be boiled or exposed to very high heat. Simmering is okay. Although cooking at high heat destroys some of its nutritional benefits, most of the flavor will remain.

Developing the recipes for this book involved my favorite kind of innovative cooking—new territory with no set rules. The following recipes are truly fusion cuisine, combining the best of east and west, making it easy to add miso to your everyday meals.

*The miso used in these recipes was made by American Miso Company. Other brands will vary in name, flavor, and nutritional content. You may have to make some minor adjustments if you use another brand.*

Notes

1. Mark Messina, Ph.D., Virginia Messina, R.D., and Kenneth D.R. Stechell, Ph.D., *The Simple Soybean and Your Health*, Avery Publishing Group, Garden City Park, N.Y., 1994, p. 120.

2. William Shurtleff and Akiko Aoyagi, *The Book of Miso*, Ten Speed Press, Berkeley, CA, 1983, pp. 25-26.

3. "Chemoprevention of N-nitroso-N-methylurea-induced Rat Mammary Cancer by Miso and Tamoxifen, Alone and in Combination," *Japan Journal Cancer Research*, Vol. 89, No. 4, May 1998, pp. 487-495.

4. "Quantification of Genistein and Genistin in Soybeans and Soybean Products," *Food Chem Toxicol*, Vol. 34, No. 5, May 1996, pp. 457-461.

# *It's Alive!!!!*

*To gain a better understanding of how miso is made, I visited the American Miso Company in North Carolina for a few days to observe the process. American Miso is the largest miso manufacturer in the world using the traditional Japanese methods. Their location in the foothills of the Smoky Mountains provides climatic conditions similar to some regions of Japan. At least six different types of miso are made there. For Greg, who has been running this operation for several years with the help of his brother Dave and a crew of locals, making miso has become a way of life.*

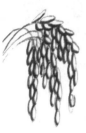

As I walked inside the high-ceiling industrial building, out of the cool, misty morning, I was wrapped in a sweet, warm, seductive aroma. This was the first morning of the three-day process for preparing the miso for fermentation. Over half of the area inside the building was filled with forty-six towering wooden vats, each one holding about 7,500 pounds of miso in varying stages of fermentation. Each vat was topped with a cover made of wooden slats that was held in place with piles of large, clean, smooth river rocks.

The sweet aroma that met me at the door was from steamed rice. It had been soaked for about an hour, then steamed, and cooled. As I walked in, the prepared rice was being combined with *aspergillus oryzae* spores. The rice was blown through a large, long horizontal tube. The spores were blown into the rice through a smaller tube connected about half way down the larger tube. The starter spores came from Japan. Originally in the traditional method, the cooked, cooled rice was tossed into the air where it mixed with the spores, which were naturally floating in the air.

The next step in the process was to spread the inoculated rice into large, flat, box-like containers set up on wheels. The containers were then wrapped in insulating blankets and rolled into a special room called the koji room to incubate overnight. Here the inoculated rice becomes what is called koji—the mycelium that produces the enzymes which transform the mixture of beans, grain, and salt into miso during fermentation.

After the koji had been put to bed to incubate, the soybeans (or in some cases chick-peas) were rinsed and left soaking in water to be ready for pressure cooking in the morning.

We inspected the koji one last time before I left for the night, feeling it for moisture and cohesiveness. We checked the temperature at the top of the room and about halfway down, and adjusted the openings in small windows in the top of the room and the door. The growing spores had to be checked about every hour, and Greg continued the vigil throughout the night.

By the next morning, the koji had grown visible short white "hairs." By midday, the grains of rice had been transformed to a pearly white and had started to turn to sugar. At that point, the rice was transferred into smaller trays. Each batch of koji was formed by hand into its own mountains and valleys to help keep the humidity consistent throughout. Then the trays went back into the koji room to incubate overnight, again being closely watched for subtle changes in temperature and humidity.

There wasn't much sleep for Greg that night. It was cold, down to about 25°F, so he spent much of the night checking the koji, and adjusting the temperature, heat, and humidity. By the next morning when I returned, the koji had become quite sweet in flavor and had grown more of its distinctive white "hairs" which were furry in texture to the tongue upon tasting. The growing of these "hairs" is essential to the process of making miso.

Even with a night of little sleep, Greg was cheery and moving quickly when I arrived at 8:30 AM on the third day. He had already started the next part of the process, which was done in batches. Depending on what type of miso is being prepared, the soybeans are either pressure steamed or pressure boiled. Steaming makes darker beans for darker miso and boiling makes lighter beans for lighter miso. That day the soybeans were pressure steamed in a large cooker, and then spread out to cool on a big stainless steel tray. They were then ground and mixed with the koji and sea salt in a large mixer.

Everything was measured out carefully so the batches could be put together in a smooth and orderly progression: tubs of koji, tubs of ground soybeans, and bags of sea salt. After each batch was mixed, it was deposited *en masse* into one of those towering wooden vats. Greg was constantly checking with his co-workers to be sure that everything was in order. This continued all day long until the vat was full. From this point, the fermentation process took its own course.

Greg told me that the fermentation process takes from one to three summers. The age of the miso is counted by summers, since that is when the microorganisms truly bloom. If you visit a miso factory, in the summer months, vats of fermenting miso may speak to you in gurgles as you walk by.

As simple as this process may seem, it demands great sensitivity and there is no substitute for experience. As with all cooking, the mental state of the cook, or miso maker in this case, has an effect on the outcome. We are the beneficiaries of this ancient process. It gives us a versatile, ready-to-use food, abundant in both nutrients and health-enhancing microorganisms with a variety of robust flavors and aromas to enrich our everyday meals.

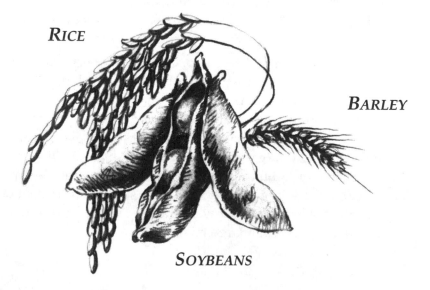

*RICE*

*BARLEY*

*SOYBEANS*

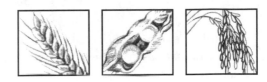

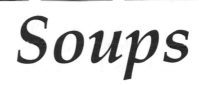

# *Soups*

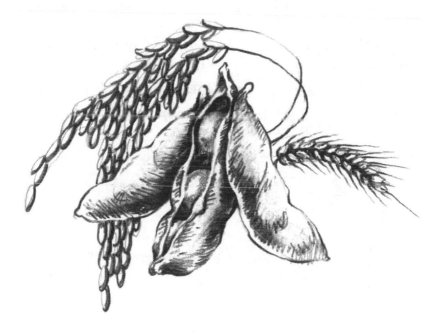

# *Onion Soup*

Yield: 4½ cups

*Blending red miso with caramelized onions adds a distinctive savory element to this classic soup. Chick-pea miso lends a sweeter, but still savory, flavor.*

> **2 cups sliced yellow onions (about ½ pound)**
> **2 tablespoons canola oil**
> **4 cups hot water**
> **3 tablespoons red miso, or 4 tablespoons**
>    **chick-pea miso**
> **⅛ teaspoon freshly ground black pepper, or to taste**

1. In a soup pot, sauté the onions in the canola oil until they are caramelized.
2. Add 3 cups of the hot water, and bring to a boil.
3. Dissolve the miso in the remaining hot water, turn off the heat, and add to the onion mixture.
4. Season to taste with the black pepper.

Per cup: Calories 97, Soy Protein 3 g, Total Protein 3 g,
Fat 6 g, Carbohydrates 7 g, Fiber 1 g, Sodium 682 mg

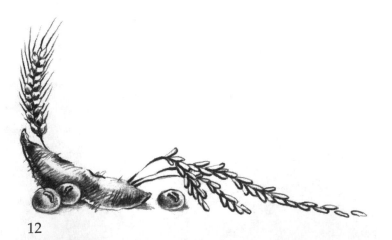

# *Vegetable Soup*

Yield: about 8 cups

*You can use any vegetables you have on hand for this soup.*

**1 medium onion, chopped**
**2 cloves garlic, minced**
**1 stalk celery, chopped**
**1 carrot, chopped**
**1 tablespoon olive oil**
**5 cups water**
**1 bay leaf**
**1 cup chopped fresh or frozen green beans**
**1 cup fresh or frozen corn**
**1 cup chopped fresh or frozen broccoli**
**1 cup green or cooked soybeans**
**2 tablespoons chopped fresh parsley**
**¼ cup sweet barley miso**

1. In a soup pot, sauté the onion, garlic, celery, and carrot in the olive oil.
2. Add the water, bay leaf, green beans, corn, broccoli, soybeans, and parsley, and simmer until the vegetables are tender.
3. Turn off the heat and stir in the miso. Serve hot with bread or crackers.

Per cup: Calories 105, Soy Protein 4 g, Total Protein 5 g,
Fat 2 g, Carbohydrates 13 g, Fiber 3 g, Sodium 329 mg

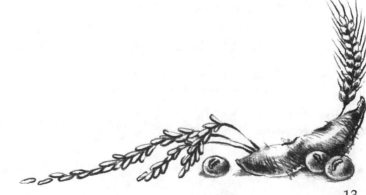

# North African Sweet Potato Soup

Yield: 16 cups

*This is a tangy, savory soup with an appealing golden color. (Pictured on the cover and opposite page 32.)*

> 8 cups vegetable stock or water
> 3 pounds sweet potatoes, peeled and thinly sliced
> 1 large onion, chopped
> 4 cloves garlic, minced
> 1 tablespoon olive oil
> 1 teaspoon cumin
> 4 teaspoons minced fresh ginger (½ ounce)
> ½ cup fresh cilantro, chopped (1 ounce)
> ¼ teaspoon cayenne
> ½ cup lime juice
> ½ cup sweet barley miso
> 2 cups hot water

1. In a soup pot, combine the stock and sweet potatoes, and simmer until tender.

2. Sauté the onion and garlic in the olive oil until transparent. Stir in the cumin and ginger, and cook for a few minutes until the cumin is slightly toasted.

3. Blend the sweet potatoes and onion mixture in a food processor or blender until smooth. Return to the soup pot, stir in the cilantro, cayenne, and lime juice, and heat to a simmer. Dissolve the miso in the hot water, and stir into the pot. Serve hot with cilantro leaf sprinkled on top.

Per cup: Calories 124, Soy Protein 2 g, Total Protein 3 g,
Fat 1 g, Carbohydrates 25 g, Fiber 3 g, Sodium 324 mg

**Variation:** In a hot oven, roast the sweet potatoes, then blend until smooth for a sweeter soup with a roasted flavor.

# Cauliflower Soup

Yield: 6 cups

*This is a delicately flavored, creamy soup with a touch of saffron.*

**2 sweet onions, chopped
4 cloves garlic, minced
1 tablespoon olive oil
1 quart water
4 cups chopped cauliflower, raw or steamed
Pinch of saffron
1 tablespoon sweet white miso
Roasted red bell pepper strips, for garnish
Chopped parsley, for garnish**

1. In a soup pot, sauté the onions and garlic in the olive oil until they start to caramelize.
2. Add the water and cauliflower. If you are using raw cauliflower, boil the soup until the cauliflower is just tender. If it has already been cooked, just heat to boiling.
3. Add the saffron.
4. Pour the soup into a food processor or blender along with the miso, and blend until smooth and creamy.
5. Return the soup to the pot, and reheat to just before boiling. Serve topped with roasted sweet red pepper strips and chopped parsley.

Per cup: Calories 61, Soy Protein 1 g, Total Protein 2 g,
Fat 2 g, Carbohydrates 8 g, Fiber 2 g, Sodium 156 mg

# Miso Kombu Soup

Yield: 8 servings

*The flavors of seaweed and miso are a classic blend. Kombu is a natural flavor enhancer containing glutamic acid. In cooking, it softens the fibers of other foods, reducing cooking time. This soup is pictured on the cover and opposite page 32.*

½ ounce kombu (about 12 inches)
6 cups water
1 carrot, cut in matchstick size pieces
6 green onions, finely sliced, including
    part of the green
½ pound spinach, baby leaves or large leaves cut
    into 1-inch strips
½ cup sweet white miso

1. Wipe any white powder off the kombu with a damp cloth. Boil it in the water for about 15 minutes. Remove the kombu. (To reuse the kombu in another broth, let it dry on a mat. Store in a covered container in the refrigerator for no more than a few days.)

2. Add the carrot and boil for 5 minutes.

3. Turn off the heat and add the green onions and spinach.

4. Dip out ½ cup of the hot broth, and mix with the miso. Continue stirring until the mixture is smooth, then pour it back into the soup pot, and stir. Do not boil. Serve immediately.

Per cup: Calories 57, Soy Protein 3 g, Total Protein 4 g,
Fat 0 g, Carbohydrates 7 g, Fiber 2 g, Sodium 896 mg

**Variation:** Add ½ pound tofu or ½ (12.3-ounce) package silken tofu cut in small cubes to the soup along with the onions and spinach.

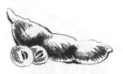

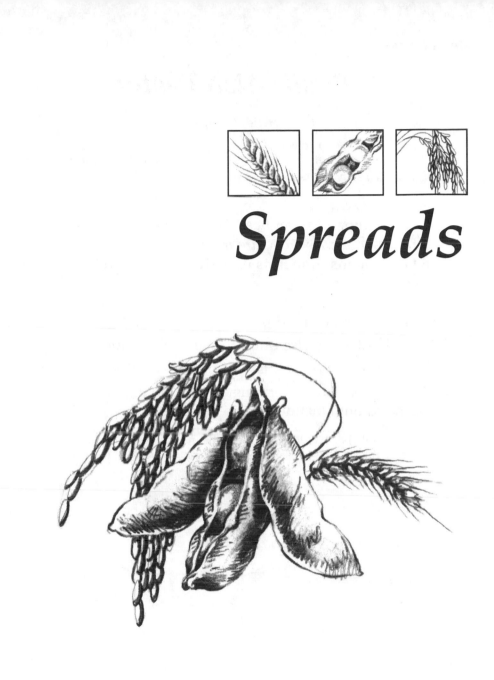

# *Spreads*

# *Basil Miso Pesto*

Yield: ⅔ cup

*Use this tasty new pesto to toss with pasta, serve as a dip for chips or vegetables, or as a salad dressing.*

**2 cloves garlic**
**3 cups chopped fresh basil (4 ounces)**
**2 tablespoons sweet white miso**
**6 tablespoons pine nuts or walnuts or a mixture**
**¼ cup olive oil**

1. Chop the garlic in a food processor.

2. Add the basil and pulse until it is coarsely chopped.

3. Add the miso and pine nuts, and process until well chopped.

4. While the processor is running, slowly pour in the olive oil, and process until blended.

Per tablespoon: Calories 95, Soy Protein 1 g, Total Protein 2 g,
Fat 7 g, Carbohydrates 3 g, Fiber 1 g, Sodium 174 mg

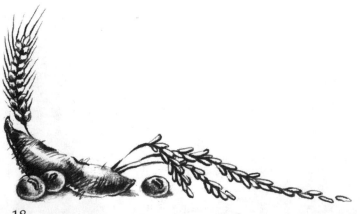

# *Cilantro Miso Pesto*

Yield: 1 cup

*From the first time I put this pesto together, it became a frequent addition to daily menus. Serve this unique and colorful pesto tossed with hot pasta or as a dip or spread for chips, crackers, or raw vegetables. You can also add a little more oil and some vinegar to make a tasty salad dressing. Hempseed has a unique nutty flavor plus all of the essential amino acids and both omega-6 and omega-3 fatty acids. You can serve this as an appetizer in bite-size pastry shells. (See the picture opposite page 33.)*

**1½ cups chopped cilantro (3 ounces)**
**2 to 4 cloves garlic**
**½ cup raw cashews or hulled hempseeds**
**2 tablespoons sweet white miso, mellow white miso**
**    or sweet barley miso**
**2 tablespoons olive oil (optional)**

1. In a food processor, chop the cilantro and garlic until minced.
2. Add the cashews, miso, and olive oil, and process until well blended.

Per tablespoon: Calories 34, Soy Protein 0 g, Total Protein 1 g,
Fat 1 g, Carbohydrates 2 g, Fiber 0 g, Sodium 111 mg

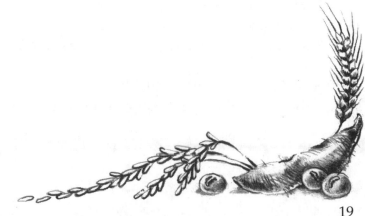

# Miso Potato Topping

Yield: about ½ cup

*Try this creamy topping on your mashed or baked potatoes in place of butter and sour cream.*

**¼ pound regular tofu**
**2 tablespoons sweet white miso**
**2 tablespoons canola oil**
**1 tablespoon fresh lemon juice**

Combine all the ingredients in a blender or food processor, and process until creamy.

Per tablespoon: Calories 53, Soy Protein 2 g, Total Protein 2 g,
Fat 3 g, Carbohydrates 2 g, Fiber 0 g, Sodium 219 mg

# Chick-Pea Spread

Yield: 1¼ cups

*This is an easy and tasty hummus with a new twist. Serve it with pita bread or as a dip with raw vegetables.*

**1 clove garlic**
**1 cup cooked chick-peas**
**2 tablespoons chick-pea or sweet white miso**
**1 tablespoon fresh lemon juice**
**2 tablespoons unsalted tahini or cashew butter**

1. Chop the garlic in a food processor.
2. Add the rest of the ingredients, and process until creamy.

Per tablespoon: Calories 29, Soy Protein 0 g, Total Protein 1 g,
Fat 0 g, Carbohydrates 3 g, Fiber 1 g, Sodium 92 mg

# Roasted Pepper Dip or Spread

Yield: 1½ cups

*Serve this colorful blend as a dip with chips or raw vegetables or as a spread with crackers. You can fill individual bite-size tarts for an eye-catching appetizer. (See the picture opposite page 33.) It can also be used as a sauce to serve with Sweet Pepper Onion Quiche (page 65). (See the picture opposite page 65.)*

**1 pound green, red, or yellow bell peppers**
**6 cloves garlic, peeled**
**1 tablespoon balsamic vinegar**
**1½ tablespoons mellow white miso**
**1 tablespoon olive oil**

1. Roast, peel, and seed the peppers.
2. Roast the garlic cloves in a hot pan until they are toasted, have a sweet aroma, and are soft.
3. Blend all the ingredients in a food processor.

Per tablespoon: Calories 13, Soy Protein 0 g, Total Protein 0 g,
Fat 0 g, Carbohydrates 1 g, Fiber 0 g, Sodium 55 mg

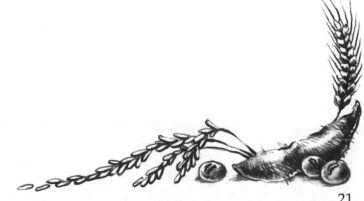

# Tofu Walnut Spread

Yield: 1½ cups

*This is a simple and tasty spread for crackers or bread, or a dip for veggies.*

**½ pound tofu**
**½ cup walnuts**
**2 tablespoons sweet white or yellow miso**

Combine all the ingredients in a food processor, and blend until creamy.

Per tablespoon: Calories 27, Soy Protein 1 g, Total Protein 1 g,
Fat 1 g, Carbohydrates 1 g, Fiber 0 g, Sodium 73 mg

# Cashew Miso Spread

Yield: about ⅔ cup

*Try this spread on crackers or bread, or use as a dip for raw vegetables.*

**¼ cup unsalted raw or roasted cashews**
**1 tablespoon sweet white miso**
**4 ounces soft tofu**

1. Finely chop the cashews in a food processor or blender.
2. Add the miso and tofu, and blend until smooth.

Per tablespoon: Calories 35, Soy Protein 1 g, Total Protein 2 g,
Fat 2 g, Carbohydrates 2 g, Fiber 0 g, Sodium 88 mg

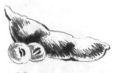

# Black-Eyed Pea Spread or Dip

Yield: 2 cups

*Try this as a dip with chips or raw vegetables, or as a burrito or taco filling. If you use canned beans that have salt, reduce the amount of miso.*

**1 clove garlic**
**¼ cup chopped onion**
**½ ounce fresh cilantro**
**1 scant cup cooked black-eyed peas, or 1 (16-ounce) can**
**1½ to 2 tablespoons mellow barley miso**
**Pinch of cayenne to taste**

1. Chop the garlic, onion, and cilantro in a food processor.

2. Add the black-eyed peas, miso, and cayenne, and blend until smooth.

Per tablespoon: Calories 9, Soy Protein 0 g, Total Protein 1 g,
Fat 0 g, Carbohydrates 1 g, Fiber 1 g, Sodium 48 mg

# Miso Walnut Spread

Yield: ¾ cup

*Try this spread on crackers or bread or as a dip for raw vegetables.*

**1 small clove garlic**
**3 tablespoons chopped walnuts (1 ounce)**
**2 tablespoons red or barley miso**
**1 tablespoon lemon juice**
**1 teaspoon liquid sweetener of choice**
**¼ cup water**
**½ cup mashed tofu (¼ pound)**

1. Chop the garlic and walnuts in a food processor or blender.
2. Add the rest of the ingredients, and blend until smooth.

Per tablespoon: Calories 26, Soy Protein 1 g, Total Protein 1 g,
Fat 1 g, Carbohydrates 1 g, Fiber 0 g, Sodium 171 mg

# White Bean Spread

Yield: 2½ cups

*I think this spread is best served hot, but can also be served cold as a spread on bread, crackers, tortillas, or raw vegetables.*

**4 cloves garlic, minced**
**1 large onion, chopped**
**1 tablespoon olive oil**
**½ tablespoon minced fresh tarragon**
**2 cups cooked white beans, or 1 (15-ounce) can**
    **unsalted beans**
**½ tablespoon Dijon mustard**
**3 tablespoons sweet white miso**

1. Sauté the garlic and onion in the olive oil until they caramelize.
2. Blend all the ingredients together in a food processor or blender until smooth.

Per tablespoon: Calories 20, Soy Protein 0 g, Total Protein 1 g,
Fat 0 g, Carbohydrates 3 g, Fiber 0 g, Sodium 98 mg

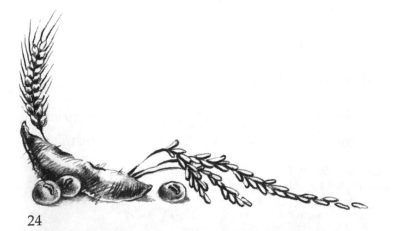

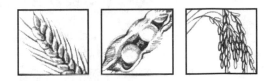

# Salads and Dressings

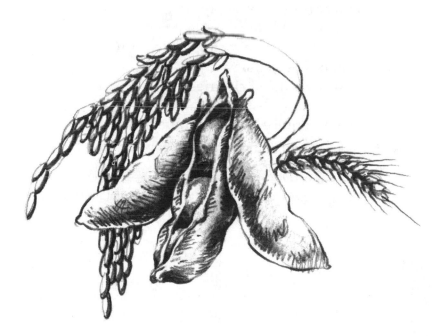

# *Apple, Celery, Cherry, and Walnut Salad*

Yield: 4 servings (4 cups)

*This salad has a tangy, sweet flavor. Make it no more than 3 hours ahead of time, cover, and chill until served.*

### *Dressing*

**2 tablespoons lemon juice**
**2 tablespoons olive oil**
**½ teaspoon Dijon mustard**
**1 tablespoon sweet white miso**

### *Salad*

**1½ cups chopped red apples**
**1½ cups chopped green apples**
**½ cup chopped celery**
**6 tablespoons coarsely chopped walnuts**
**¼ cup chopped parsley**
**2 tablespoons dried cherries**

1. Blend the lemon juice, olive oil, mustard, and miso.
2. Toss the salad ingredients together, pour the dressing over the salad, and toss again.

Per serving: Calories 228, Soy Protein 1 g, Total Protein 3 g,
Fat 13 g, Carbohydrates 24 g, Fiber 5 g, Sodium 232 mg

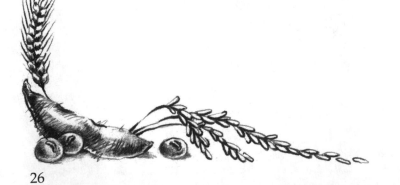

# Asian Greek Salad

Yield: 6 to 8 servings

*This salad combines Asian, Greek, and south-of-the-border flavors. This recipe is from* Soyfoods Cookery.

## Dressing

¼ cup olive oil
2 tablespoons wine vinegar
2 tablespoons mellow white miso
¼ teaspoon freshly ground black pepper
2 cloves garlic
2 tablespoons minced fresh basil
1 tablespoon minced fresh oregano

1 pound firm tofu, cut into ½-inch cubes
1 head leaf lettuce
2 fresh tomatoes, chopped
2 cucumbers, cubed
1 avocado, cubed
½ small red onion, chopped
½ cup Greek or black olives

1. Combine the olive oil, vinegar, miso, black pepper, and garlic and mix. Stir in the basil and oregano.
2. Pour the dressing over the tofu cubes in a glass or stainless steel bowl, and marinate for at least 1 hour or overnight.
3. Break the lettuce leaves apart, then wash and dry the lettuce. Arrange in a salad bowl.
4. In a separate bowl, toss the marinated tofu and all the rest of the ingredients together. Serve in the lettuce lined bowl.

Per serving: Calories 223, Soy Protein 5 g, Total Protein 7 g,
Fat 15 g, Carbohydrates 12 g, Fiber 4 g, Sodium 429 mg

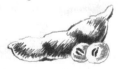

# Cabbage Peanut Slaw

Yield: 6 cups

*With a tang and a bit of ginger, this flavorful slaw will add flair to a meal.*

### Dressing
½ teaspoon grated fresh ginger
3 tablespoons chopped fresh cilantro leaves (¼ ounce)
¼ cup rice vinegar
1 tablespoon sesame oil
2 tablespoons mellow white miso
1 teaspoon sweetener of choice

### Salad
½ pound snow peas, stringed and sliced diagonally
½ pound napa or savoy cabbage, shredded
6 green onions, chopped (use part of the green)
1 medium carrot, shredded (about 1 cup), or 1 medium
    red bell pepper, chopped
¼ cup chopped peanuts

1. In a blender, chop the ginger and cilantro leaves. Add the rest of the dressing ingredients, and blend.
2. Toss all the salad ingredients together, pour the dressing over them, and toss again.

Per cup: Calories 110, Soy Protein 1 g, Total Protein 4 g,
Fat 5 g, Carbohydrates 11 g, Fiber 4 g, Sodium 416 mg

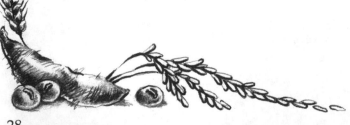

# Edamame Salad

Yield: 10 servings (5 cups)

**1 pound shelled frozen or fresh edamame
(about 4½ cups)
1 red bell pepper, chopped
1 recipe Basil Salad Dressing (page 39)**

1. Steam or boil frozen edamame for 7 to 8 minutes (fresh for 20 minutes) until tender.
2. Toss all the ingredients together, chill, and serve.

Per serving: Calories 99, Soy Protein 5 g, Total Protein 5 g,
Fat 5 g, Carbohydrates 7 g, Fiber 2 g, Sodium 88 mg

# Green Pea Salad

Yield: 10 servings (5 cups)

**1 pound shelled fresh or frozen peas (about 4½ cups)
1 red bell pepper, chopped
1 recipe Mustard-Miso Vinaigrette (page 37)**

1. Steam or boil the peas for 5 to 7 minutes until tender.
2. Toss all the ingredients together, chill, and serve.

Per serving: Calories 91, Soy Protein 2 g, Total Protein 2 g,
Fat 6 g, Carbohydrates 7 g, Fiber 2 g, Sodium 184 mg

# Orange, Jicama, and Avocado Salad with Sweet Mustard Vinaigrette

Yield: 4 servings

*Tangy, sweet and sour, this salad will stand out at any meal.*

### Sweet Mustard Vinaigrette

> 2 tablespoons red wine vinegar
> 2 tablespoons olive oil
> 1½ tablespoons sweet white miso
> 1 tablespoon Dijon mustard
> 1 tablespoon sweetener of choice
> 2 teaspoons organic orange zest

### Salad

> 4 ounces baby lettuce
> 2 oranges, peeled and sectioned
> ¼ pound jicama, cut into matchsticks
> 1 ripe avocado, peeled and thinly sliced

1. Combine all the dressing ingredients in a blender, or mix in a bowl with a whip.
2. On separate plates, arrange equal parts of the lettuce, orange sections, jicama, and avocado.
3. Pour 2 tablespoons of the dressing over each salad.

Per serving: Calories 230, Soy Protein 1 g, Total Protein 3 g, Fat 13 g, Carbohydrates 23 g, Fiber 4 g, Sodium 380 mg

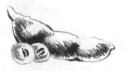

# Pear and Cherry Salad

Yield: 4 servings

*For a slightly different flavor, try lightly grilling the sliced pears. The tangy herb dressing adds just the right finishing touch. (See the picture opposite page 65.)*

## Dressing

**2 tablespoons sweet white miso**
**1 tablespoon olive oil**
**2 tablespoons raspberry, mango, or apple cider vinegar**
**1 tablespoon liquid sweetener of choice**
**3 tablespoons chopped fresh basil (¼ ounce)**
**3 tablespoons chopped fresh parsley (¼ ounce)**

## Salad

**About 4 ounces mesclun salad greens**
**1 pear, thinly sliced lengthwise**
**2 ounces dried cherries**
**2 ounces walnuts, broken**
**Fresh raspberries, for garnish (optional)**

1. Combine the dressing ingredients in a blender or food processor.
2. On individual plates, make a bed of the mesclun salad greens.
3. Fan some of the pear slices over each plate of lettuce, and sprinkle on the dried cherries and walnuts.
4. Drizzle 2 tablespoons of dressing per serving over the salad. Top each salad with a few raspberries.

Per serving: Calories218 , Soy Protein 2 g, Total Protein 4 g,
Fat 11 g, Carbohydrates 21 g, Fiber 3 g, Sodium 440 mg

# George Washington Carver Memorial Sweet Potato Salad

Yield: 6 servings (6 cups)

*Although he probably did not have miso, Dr. Carver was one of the early proponents of using soybeans as "people food" in the West. Around the turn of the twentieth century, his research demonstrated that soybeans are a valuable source of protein and oil. This unique and colorful salad blends three of Dr. Carver's focus foods—sweet potatoes, peanuts, and soybeans.*

**2 pounds sweet potatoes, peeled and cubed
(about 5½ cups)
¾ cup Tofu Mayo (page 39)
½ cup chopped peanuts
½ cup chopped fresh cilantro
½ cup chopped green onions (use part of the green)**

1. Steam the sweet potatoes until they are tender but not mushy. Remove from the heat and allow to cool.

2. Toss the sweet potatoes with all of the other ingredients, and chill.

Per serving: Calories 258, Soy Protein 3 g, Total Protein 7 g,
Fat 6 g, Carbohydrates 41 g, Fiber 7 g, Sodium 279 mg

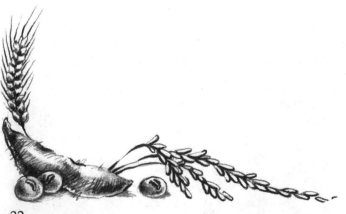

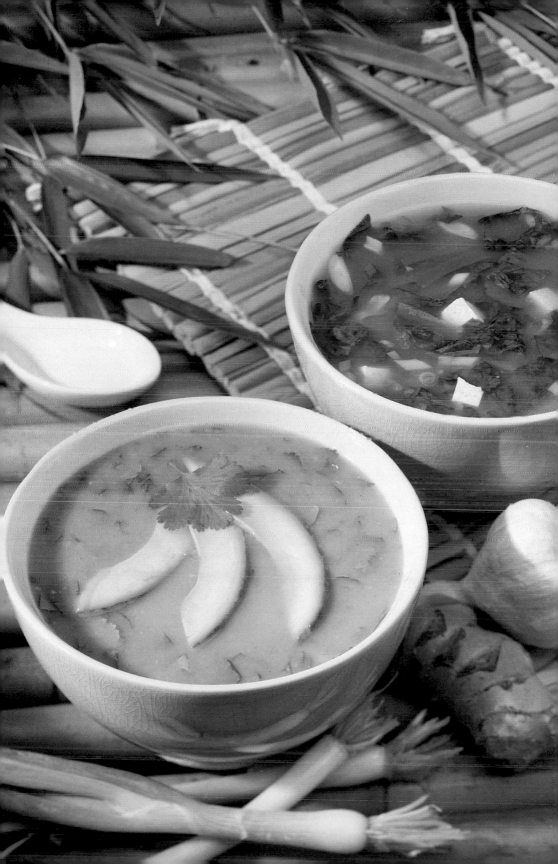

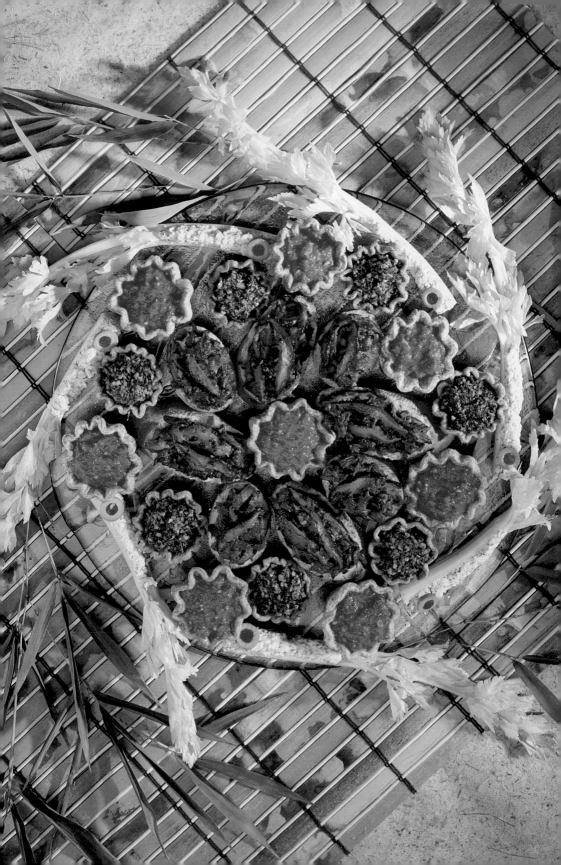

# Spinach Salad with Marinated Tofu

Yield: 4 servings

*This salad can be started the day before by marinating the tofu overnight in its special dressing. If you can't find baby spinach leaves, try a bed of mesclun.*

## Dressing

    **1 clove garlic**
    **2 tablespoons sweet white miso**
    **1½ tablespoons mirin**
    **2 tablespoons fresh lemon juice**
    **½ teaspoon basil**
    **¼ teaspoon oregano**

    **½ pound tofu, cut into ½-inch cubes**
    **½ pound baby spinach leaves**
    **¼ red onion, thinly sliced**

1. Chop the garlic in a small blender, add the miso, mirin, lemon juice, basil, and oregano, and blend until smooth.
2. Pour the dressing over the tofu, and toss carefully. Cover and refrigerate to marinate overnight.
3. Serve on a bed of fresh baby spinach, and garnish with the red onion slices.

Per serving: Calories 163, Soy Protein 7 g, Total Protein 9 g, Fat 3 g, Carbohydrates 19 g, Fiber 3 g, Sodium 780 mg

# Roasted Vegetable Salad with Chick-Peas

Yield: 4 servings (6 cups)

*Roasted vegetables make a flavorful salad. Add chick-peas for protein and toss with this zesty herbed miso dressing for a satisfying one-dish meal.*

## Salad

1½ pounds summer squash and zucchini,
 sliced ¼ inch thick
1 small red bell pepper, cut into 1-inch pieces
1 small yellow bell pepper, cut into 1-inch pieces
1 small orange bell pepper, cut into 1-inch pieces
1 small onion, cut in 1-inch pieces
1 clove garlic
3 tablespoons chopped fresh basil (¼ ounce)
1 tablespoon olive oil
2 cups cooked chick-peas, or 1 (15-ounce) can
 unsalted chick-peas

## Dressing

3 tablespoons mellow white miso
1 tablespoon olive oil
2 tablespoons balsamic vinegar
3 tablespoons chopped fresh basil (¼ ounce)
3 tablespoons chopped fresh parsley (¼ ounce)
1 clove garlic, minced

Red or yellow cherry tomatoes, for garnish

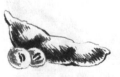

1. Preheat the oven to 450°F.

2. Toss the squash, peppers, onion, garlic, and basil with the 1 tablespoon olive oil, and spread out on a baking sheet. Roast in the oven for 15 to 20 minutes, or until tender when pricked with a fork.

3. In a bowl, toss the vegetables together with the chick-peas.

4. Blend the dressing ingredients and pour over the vegetable/chick-pea mix, toss, and chill. Marinate for several hours or overnight.

5. Serve on a bed of lettuce and garnish with red or yellow cherry tomatoes.

Per serving: Calories 280, Soy Protein 2 g, Total Protein 11 g,
Fat 8 g, Carbohydrates 38 g, Fiber 8 g, Sodium 915 mg

*Variation:* Replace the chick-peas with 1 pound firm tofu cut into ¾-inch cubes.

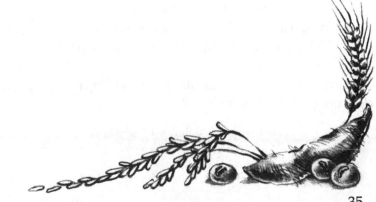

# Cole Slaw Dressing with Soy Protein Isolate

Yield: about 1½ cups

*This makes a creamy, tangy dressing for your favorite slaw combination.*

**1 clove garlic, minced**
**½ cup olive oil**
**½ cup apple cider vinegar**
**¼ cup sweetener of choice**
**¼ cup soy protein isolate**
**1 tablespoon mellow barley miso**
**1 very small or ¼ medium onion, chopped (1 ounce)**

Combine all the ingredients in a blender until smooth.

Per tablespoon: Calories 58, Soy Protein 1 g, Total Protein 1 g,
Fat 4 g, Carbohydrates 4 g, Fiber 0 g, Sodium 48 mg

# Creamy Tofu Cole Slaw Dressing

Yield: about 2 cups

**1 (12.3-ounce) package silken tofu**
**4 tablespoons apple cider or rice vinegar**
**4 tablespoons sweet white miso**
**1 tablespoon sweetener of choice**
**½ to 1 teaspoon garlic powder, or 1 clove garlic, minced**
**¼ teaspoon freshly ground black pepper**

Combine all the ingredients in a blender or food processor until smooth and creamy.

Per tablespoon: Calories 15, Soy Protein 1 g, Total Protein 1 g,
Fat 0 g, Carbohydrates 2 g, Fiber 0 g, Sodium 112 mg

# Creamy Ginger Sesame Dressing

Yield: about ¾ cup

*This dressing has just the right bite of ginger and garlic for your salad.*

**2 teaspoons minced fresh ginger (¼ ounce)**
**1 clove garlic**
**¼ cup rice vinegar**
**2 tablespoons sweet white miso**
**2 tablespoons mirin**
**2 tablespoons sesame oil**
**¼ cup mashed tofu**
**1 tablespoon sesame seeds**

1. Chop the ginger and garlic in a blender or small food processor.
2. Add the rest of the ingredients, and blend until creamy.

Per tablespoon: Calories 54, Soy Protein 1 g, Total Protein 1 g,
Fat 2 g, Carbohydrates 5 g, Fiber 0 g, Sodium 190 mg

# Mustard-Miso Vinaigrette

Yield: ⅔ cup

*This is a full-bodied dressing.*

**1 clove garlic**
**1 tablespoon Dijon or stone-ground mustard**
**2 tablespoons balsamic vinegar**
**1 tablespoon brown rice or red miso**
**¼ cup olive oil**
**2 tablespoons water**

1. Chop the garlic in a blender.
2. Add the rest of the ingredients, and blend well.

Per tablespoon: Calories 53, Soy Protein 0 g, Total Protein 0 g,
Fat 6 g, Carbohydrates 0 g, Fiber 0 g, Sodium 144 mg

# Sweet-Salty Salad Dressing

Yield: about 2 cups

*This is a good dressing for a green salad with citrus.*

**2 cloves garlic**
**1 tablespoon mellow barley miso**
**½ cup olive oil**
**½ cup apple cider vinegar**
**½ cup soymilk**
**¼ cup liquid sweetener of choice**

Combine all the ingredients in a blender until smooth.

Per tablespoon: Calories 42, Soy Protein 0 g, Total Protein 0 g,
Fat 2 g, Carbohydrates 2 g, Fiber 0 g, Sodium 28 mg

# Sweet Miso Mustard Dressing or Dip

Yield: ¾ cup

*Serve this with salad as a dressing or as a dip with raw vegetables*

**¼ cup sweet white miso**
**¼ cup rice vinegar**
**2 tablespoons soy oil**
**1 tablespoon liquid sweetener of choice**
**¼ teaspoon dry mustard**

Combine all the ingredients in a blender until smooth and creamy.

Per tablespoon: Calories 42, Soy Protein 1 g, Total Protein 1 g,
Fat 2 g, Carbohydrates 3 g, Fiber 0 g, Sodium 290 mg

# Basil Salad Dressing

Yield: ⅓ cup

1 clove garlic
6 tablespoons chopped fresh basil (½ ounce)
1 tablespoon sweet white miso
2 tablespoons raspberry vinegar
1 teaspoon liquid sweetener of choice
2 tablespoons olive oil

1. Chop the garlic and basil in a food processor.
2. Add the rest of the ingredients, and blend.

Per tablespoon: Calories 63, Soy Protein 1 g, Total Protein 1 g,
Fat 6 g, Carbohydrates 2 g, Fiber 0 g, Sodium 174 mg

# Tofu Mayo

Yield: 1¾ cups

*Add a unique zip to your sandwich or salad with this creamy dressing.*

1 (12.3-ounce) package silken tofu
3 tablespoons apple cider vinegar or lemon juice
4 tablespoons sweet white miso, or 3 tablespoons
    red miso
½ teaspoon garlic powder
¼ teaspoon dry mustard

Combine all the ingredients in a blender until smooth and creamy.

Per tablespoon: Calories 14, Soy Protein 1 g, Total Protein 1 g,
Fat 0 g, Carbohydrates 1 g, Fiber 0 g, Sodium 129 mg

# Peanut Dressing

Yield: ⅔ cup

*This is a tasty Thai-inspired dressing for salads or dipping vegetables.*

**¼ cup peanuts**
**2 tablespoons chopped fresh cilantro (¼ ounce)**
**2 teaspoons minced fresh ginger (¼ ounce)**
**2 tablespoons sweet white miso**
**¼ cup rice vinegar**
**2 tablespoons mirin**

1. In a small food processor or blender, chop the peanuts, cilantro, and ginger.
2. Add the miso, vinegar, and mirin, and process until well blended.

Per tablespoon: Calories 53, Soy Protein 1 g, Total Protein 1 g,
Fat 2 g, Carbohydrates 6 g, Fiber 0 g, Sodium 229 mg

*Variation:* Add 4 ounces tofu and blend.

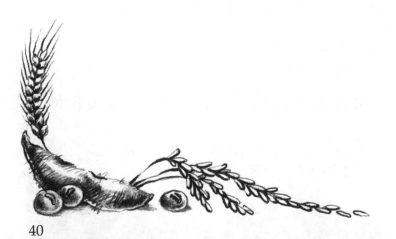

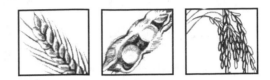

# *Sauces and Gravies*

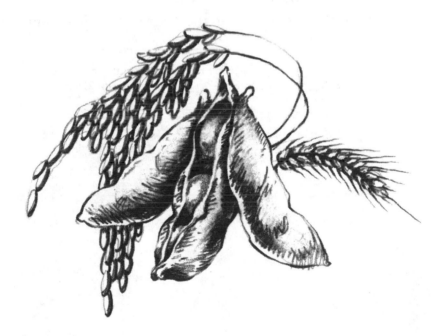

# *Apricot-Lime BBQ Sauce*

Yield: about 2 cups

*Try this with grilled tempeh or tofu.*

**⅓ cup boiling water**
**1 ounce dried apricots, chopped**
**¼ cup lime juice**
**2 tablespoons mellow barley miso**
**⅓ cup liquid sweetener of choice**
**2 cloves garlic**
**Slice of onion**
**Pinch of cayenne**

1. Pour the boiling water over the apricots, and let stand until plumped and most of the water is absorbed.

2. Thoroughly combine all of the ingredients in small food processor or blender.

Per ¼ cup: Calories 62, Soy Protein 1 g, Total Protein 1 g,
Fat 0 g, Carbohydrates 14 g, Fiber 0 g, Sodium 218 mg

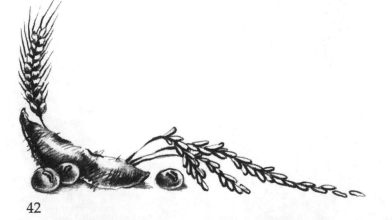

# Old Time Barbecue Sauce

Yield: 3½ cups

*Try this tangy, spicy sauce with Tofu Ribs (page 78) or cooked soybeans.*

1 medium onion, minced
2 cloves garlic, minced
1 tablespoon olive oil
1 medium green bell pepper, minced
1 (6-ounce) can tomato paste
1¼ cups water
½ cup brown sugar
¼ cup salad mustard
½ teaspoon allspice
¼ teaspoon chipotle, or to taste
2 tablespoons vinegar
2 tablespoons red or barley miso
¼ cup hot water

1. In a saucepan, sauté the onion and garlic in the olive oil.
2. Stir in the rest of the ingredients, except the miso and ¼ cup hot water, and bring to a boil. Reduce the heat and let simmer for about 10 minutes.
3. Dissolve the miso in the ¼ cup hot water. Turn off the heat and stir the miso into the sauce.

Per ¼ cup: Calories 151, Soy Protein 0 g, Total Protein 1 g,
Fat 1 g, Carbohydrates 9 g, Fiber 1 g, Sodium 207 mg

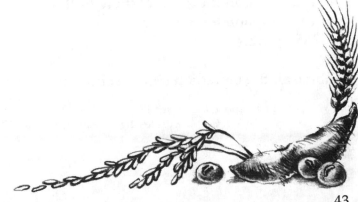

# Lemon-Basil Sauce

Yield: ¾ cup

*Top steamed vegetables with this sauce. It is especially good on steamed beets.*

**3 tablespoons chopped fresh basil or parsley (¼ ounce)**
**1 clove garlic**
**½ cup crumbled soft silken tofu**
**3 tablespoons lemon juice**
**½ teaspoon lemon zest**
**2 tablespoons sweet white miso**

1. Chop the basil and garlic in a small food processor.
2. Add the rest of the ingredients, and blend until smooth.

Per 2 tablespoons: Calories 32, Soy Protein 3 g, Total Protein 3 g,
Fat 1 g, Carbohydrates 3 g, Fiber 0 g, Sodium 298 mg

# Topping for Steamed Vegetables

Yield: about ½ cup

*Toss steamed vegetables with this topping in place of butter.*

**2 tablespoons mellow white miso**
**1 tablespoon unsalted cashew butter**
**1 tablespoon lemon juice**
**¼ cup water**

Combine all the ingredients in a blender until smooth.

Per 2 tablespoons: Calories 47, Soy Protein 2 g, Total Protein 6 g,
Fat 1 g, Carbohydrates 4 g, Fiber 0 g, Sodium 601 mg

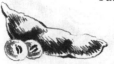

# Jerk Sauce

Yield: 1 cup

*This sauce can be used as a dip or for Jerk Tofu (page 66). Make it as hot as you like.*

**2 cloves garlic**
**½ Scotch bonnet, habañero, or other hot chile of choice, or ⅛ teaspoon cayenne**
**1 small onion**
**2 to 3 tablespoons minced fresh ginger**
**1 teaspoon allspice**
**½ teaspoon thyme**
**¼ teaspoon cinnamon**
**Pinch of nutmeg**
**2 tablespoons red miso**
**¼ cup fresh lime juice**
**¼ cup sweetener of choice**

1. Chop the garlic, pepper, onion, and ginger in a food processor.
2. Add the rest of the ingredients, and process until well blended.

Per 2 tablespoons: Calories 45, Soy Protein 1 g, Total Protein 1 g,
Fat 0 g, Carbohydrates 10 g, Fiber 0 g, Sodium 256 mg

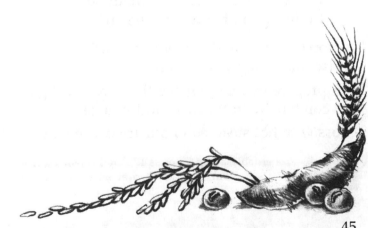

# Tofu Alfredo Sauce for Pasta

Yield: about 1¼ cups

*This creamy blend makes enough sauce for about ½ pound of uncooked pasta. Toss the sauce with the pasta while it is still hot.*

**2 cloves garlic**
**6 tablespoons chopped fresh basil (½ ounce), or**
  **1 tablespoon dried basil**
**3 tablespoons mellow white miso**
**½ pound soft tofu**

1. Chop the garlic and basil in a food processor or blender.

2. Add the miso and tofu, and blend until creamy.

Per ¼ cup: Calories 91, Soy Protein 8 g, Total Protein 8 g,
Fat 2 g, Carbohydrates 8 g, Fiber 1 g, Sodium 1226 mg

**Variation:** Use fresh cilantro leaves in place of the basil.

# Veggie Toss Sauce

Yield: 2 servings (about 3 tablespoons)

*This sauce will be enough for about 1 pound of vegetables.*

**1 clove garlic**
**1 tablespoon minced fresh ginger**
**1 tablespoon mellow white miso**
**1 tablespoon balsamic vinegar**

1. Chop the garlic and ginger in a small food processor. Add the miso and vinegar, and blend.

2. To prepare by hand, mince the garlic and ginger. Use a fork to combine with the miso and vinegar.

3. Toss with hot steamed or stir-fried vegetables, and serve.

Per tablespoon: Calories 17, Soy Protein 1 g, Total Protein 1 g,
Fat 0 g, Carbohydrates 2 g, Fiber 0 g, Sodium 400 mg

# West African Peanut Tomato Sauce

Yield: 4½ cups

*This is a variation of a classic West African sauce for pouring over steamed root vegetables. Try this sauce over a combination of carrots, sweet potatoes, and/or green beans.*

**2 onions, chopped**
**1 green bell pepper, chopped**
**4 cloves garlic, minced**
**1 teaspoon canola or peanut oil**
**1 (28-ounce) can peeled tomatoes, drained**
**(reserve the juice)**
**6 tablespoons unsalted peanut butter**
**½ teaspoon allspice**
**½ teaspoon thyme**
**⅛ teaspoon cayenne, or to taste**
**1 tablespoon red miso, or 2 tablespoons mellow white**
**miso**
**¼ cup hot water**

1. Sauté the onion, green pepper, and garlic in the oil.
2. Blend the reserved canned tomato water with the peanut butter in a blender or food processor until smooth.
3. Add the sautéed vegetables, tomatoes, allspice, thyme, and cayenne, and purée.
4. Pour this mixture into a saucepan, and simmer over low heat for about 5 minutes. Turn off the heat.
5. Dissolve the miso in the hot water, and add to the saucepan. Pour over steamed vegetables.

Per ¼ cup: Calories 50, Soy Protein 0 g, Total Protein 2 g,
Fat 2 g, Carbohydrates 4 g, Fiber 2 g, Sodium 3 mg

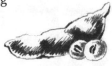

# Ginger Miso Topping

Yield: ⅓ cup

*Try tossing this topping with pasta or steamed vegetables. This is enough topping for about ¼ pound of cooked pasta.*

**1 tablespoon minced fresh ginger**
**1 clove garlic, minced**
**2 tablespoons fresh lemon juice**
**2 tablespoons olive oil**
**1½ tablespoons sweet white miso**
**Pinch of cayenne**

Combine all the ingredients in a small blender, or mix with a wire whip or fork.

Per tablespoon: Calories 63, Soy Protein 1 g, Total Protein 1 g,
Fat 5 g, Carbohydrates 2 g, Fiber 0 g, Sodium 261 mg

# Béchamel Sauce

Yield: 1¼ cups

*This is a basic béchamel with a new, rich flavor.*

**2 tablespoons oil**
**2 tablespoons unbleached white flour**
**1 cup soymilk**
**2 tablespoons sweet white miso**

1. Combine the oil and flour in a saucepan over medium heat. Let them bubble together until the flour starts to brown.
2. Whisk in ¾ cup of the soymilk until smooth. Continue to cook until the sauce thickens. Turn off the heat.
3. Whip the miso into the remaining soymilk, then whip into the cooked sauce.

Per 2 tablespoons: Calories 46, Soy Protein 1 g, Total Protein 1 g,
Fat 3 g, Carbohydrates 2 g, Fiber 0 g, Sodium 177 mg

# Kebab Sauce or Sweet and Sour Sauce

Yield: about 1 cup

*This tangy sauce can be used as a marinade for kebabs (see below) or a dipping sauce.*

**¾ cup apple or pineapple juice**
**3 tablespoons apple cider vinegar**
**2 tablespoons sweetener of choice**
**1 tablespoon grated fresh ginger**
**2 cloves garlic, minced**
**1 tablespoon cornnstarch**
**⅛ teaspoon cracked red pepper (optional)**

**2 teaspoons red or barley miso**

1. In a saucepan, whip together all the ingredients except the miso. Bring to a boil, reduce the heat to low, and cook for about 10 minutes until it thickens slightly, stirring constantly to avoid lumps. Turn off the heat.

2. Whip the miso into the sauce.

Per 2 tablespoons: Calories 34, Soy Protein 0 g, Total Protein 0 g, Fat 0 g, Carbohydrates 8 g, Fiber 0 g, Sodium 86 mg

***For Kebabs:*** Reconstitute 1½ cups (3 ounces) textured soy protein chunks in 1½ cups boiling water. Carefully squeeze dry and add to the Kebab Sauce in the saucepan along with chunks of bell pepper, zucchini, onion, and pineapple. Let marinate for a few hours, slide on to kebab sticks, and then grill.

# Hempseed Oil Garlic Sauce

Yield: 6 tablespoons

*Try this as a topping for steamed vegetables, pasta, or bread. Hempseed oil has a unique nutty flavor plus the nutritional benefits of both omega-6 and omega-3 fatty acids.*

**1 clove garlic, minced or pressed**
**¼ cup hempseed oil**
**2 tablespoons sweet white miso**

Beat all the ingredients together with a mini food processor or by hand.

Per tablespoon: Calories 95, Soy Protein 1 g, Total Protein 1 g, Fat 9 g, Carbohydrates 2 g, Fiber 0 g, Sodium 290 mg

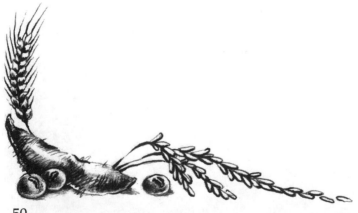

# Creamy Country Gravy

Yield: about 3 cups

*Get the biscuits ready for this creamy country style gravy with a rich flavor.*

**2 tablespoons oil**
**¼ cup unbleached flour**
**2 tablespoons nutritional yeast (optional)**
**2½ cups soymilk**
**2 tablespoons dark barley or red miso**
**1 teaspoon poultry seasoning**

1. Combine the oil, flour, and nutritional yeast in a saucepan over medium heat. Let it bubble together for a few minutes until it smells toasted and looks browned.

2. Combine the soymilk, miso, and poultry seasoning in a blender or mix with a hand blender. Whip into the toasted mixture in the saucepan, and heat to just before boiling. Do not boil. Remove any lumps with a whip or hand-held blender. Serve over Mashed Potatoes (page 57).

Per ¼ cup: Calories 50, Soy Protein 2 g, Total Protein 2 g,
Fat 3 g, Carbohydrates 3 g, Fiber 6 g, Sodium 176 mg

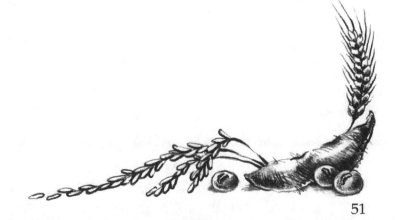

# Miso Gravy

Yield: 2¼ cups

*This hearty, savory gravy can team up with a variety of thirsty foods.*

**2 tablespoons oil**
**¼ cup unbleached flour**
**2 tablespoons nutritional yeast**
**1 tablespoon onion powder**
**1 teaspoon garlic powder**
**2 cups hot water**
**2 tablespoons red or barley miso, or to taste**

1. In a saucepan, whip together the oil, flour, and nutritional yeast. Heat until it begins to brown. Stir in the onion and garlic powder.

2. Whip in 1½ cups of the hot water until it forms a thick, smooth gravy.

3. Dissolve the miso in the remaining ½ cup hot water. Turn off the heat and whip the miso mixture into the gravy. Serve hot.

Per ¼ cup: Calories 50, Soy Protein 1 g, Total Protein 2 g,
Fat 3 g, Carbohydrates 4 g, Fiber 0 g, Sodium 229 mg

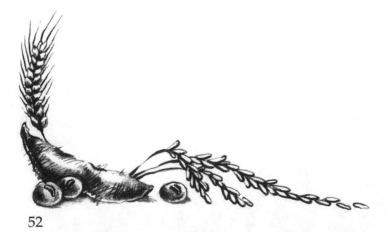

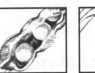

# *Vegetables*

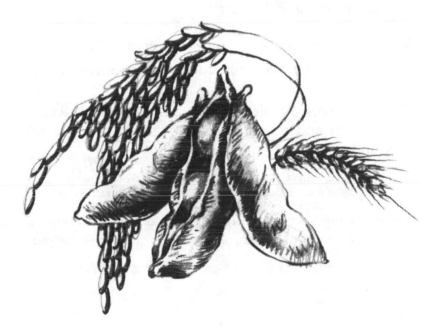

# Braised Savoy Cabbage

Yield: 4 to 6 servings (about 4 cups)

*Cabbage prepared like this will be a welcome accompaniment to any meal.*

**1 medium onion, sliced**
**3 cloves garlic, minced**
**1 tablespoon olive oil**
**4 cups shredded savoy cabbage (12 ounces)**
**½ teaspoon dried dill**
**¼ cup chopped fresh parsley**
**1 tablespoon sweet barley miso**
**3 tablespoons hot water**

1. Sauté the onion and garlic in the olive oil.
2. Add the cabbage and dill, cover, and simmer for about 8 minutes.
3. Stir in the parsley. Dissolve the miso in the hot water. Turn off the heat and pour the miso over the cabbage mixture, toss, and serve.

Per serving: Calories 82, Soy Protein 1 g, Total Protein 2 g,
Fat 4 g, Carbohydrates 9 g, Fiber 2 g, Sodium 197 mg

*Variation:* Sauté 3 ounces fresh, sliced shiitake mushrooms, or other fresh mushrooms of choice, or 2 roasted, sliced bell peppers.

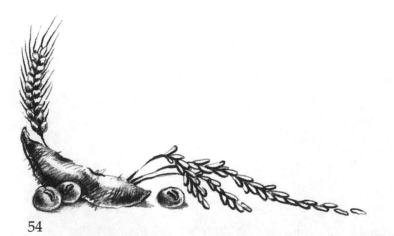

# Crispy Crunchy Sweet Pepper Stir Fry

Yield: 4 servings

*Have all the ingredients cut and ready to go before you start this eye-catching dish. Try this with Marinated Tempeh Sticks (page 64). (Pictured on the cover and opposite page 64.)*

**2 cloves garlic**
**4 teaspoons minced fresh ginger (½ ounce)**
**2 carrots, thinly sliced diagonally**
**1 tablespoon olive oil**
**6 green onions, chopped**
**1 red bell pepper, cut in triangles**
**1 yellow bell pepper, cut in triangles**
**½ pound snow peas**
**6 tablespoons chopped fresh basil (½ ounce)**
**2 tablespoons mellow white miso**
**1 tablespoon mirin**

1. Sauté the garlic, ginger, and carrots in the olive oil for about 5 minutes, covered.
2. Stir in the onions, bell peppers, peas, and basil, cover, and sauté 2 more minutes. Turn off the heat.
3. Mix the miso and mirin together, toss with the vegetables, and serve.

Per serving: Calories 173, Soy Protein 2 g, Total Protein 4 g, Fat 5 g, Carbohydrates 25 g, Fiber 6 g, Sodium 911 mg

# Green Beans with Roasted Garlic

Yield: 3 to 4 servings

*These tasty green beans are pictured on the back cover.*

**1 head garlic**
**1 tablespoon sweet or mellow barley miso**
**2 tablespoons water**
**½ tablespoon olive oil**
**1 pound small, fresh green beans, washed and trimmed**

1. Preheat the oven to 400°F.
2. Wrap the garlic head in foil or place in a garlic roaster, and bake until tender, about 20 to 30 minutes.
3. Pop off the garlic skins. In a small food processor or blender, combine the roasted garlic, miso, water, and olive oil until smooth and creamy.
4. Steam the green beans until tender, about 8 minutes.
5. Toss the green beans with the roasted garlic mixture to taste.

Per serving: Calories 70, Soy Protein 1 g, Total Protein 3 g,
Fat 1 g, Carbohydrates 10 g, Fiber 3 g, Sodium 187 mg

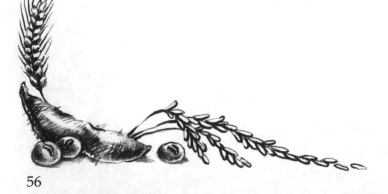

# Corn on the Cob

Yield: 8 to 10 servings

*This is a different way to "butter" your corn. (Pictured on the back cover.)*

**2 tablespoons olive oil**
**1 tablespoon sweet white miso, or**
    **½ tablespoon dark red miso**
**1 clove garlic (optional)**
**8 to 10 ears of corn, steamed, boiled, or roasted**

1. Combine the olive oil, miso, and garlic in a small blender.
2. Brush or spread on the cooked corn.

Per serving: Calories 90, Soy Protein 0 g, Total Protein 2 g,
Fat 3 g, Carbohydrates 13 g, Fiber 4 g, Sodium 100 mg

# Mashed Potatoes

Yield: 3 to 4 servings

*These unique mashed potatoes are pictured on the back cover.*

**¾ cup water**
**1½ tablespoons non-hydrogenated margarine**
**¾ cup soymilk**
**1 tablespoon mellow white or mellow barley miso**
**1 cup instant potato flakes**

1. Bring the water to a boil, add the margarine and soymilk, and reheat to almost boiling. Turn off the heat.
2. Whip in the miso and then the potato flakes with a fork until they are the consistency of mashed potatoes. Serve hot with Miso Gravy (page 52).

Per serving: Calories 279, Soy Protein 2 g, Total Protein 5 g,
Fat 6 g, Carbohydrates 50 g, Fiber 10 g, Sodium 485 mg

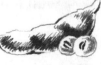

# Roasted Zucchini Rounds

Yield: 4 servings

*Toast these in the oven or pop them on the grill with your veggie burgers.*

**1 clove garlic, minced**
**3 tablespoons chopped fresh basil (¼ ounce)**
**1 tablespoon sweet white miso**
**1 tablespoon wine vinegar**
**1 tablespoon olive oil**
**2 pounds zucchini, cut into ½-inch rounds**

1. Preheat the oven to 450°F.
2. Chop the garlic and basil in a food processor. Add the miso, vinegar, and olive oil, and process until blended.
3. Toss the zucchini rounds in the miso mixture, and spread out on an oiled baking sheet. Bake for 20 minutes.

Per serving: Calories 73, Soy Protein 2 g, Total Protein 1 g,
Fat 2 g, Carbohydrates 7 g, Fiber 2 g, Sodium 224 mg

# Stuffed Celery

Yield: 1 cup stuffing

*Serve stuffed celery as an appetizer or as a side dish with soup or sandwiches. (See the picture opposite page 33.)*

**1 clove garlic**
**½ pound tofu**
**2 tablespoons mellow barley miso**
**1 tablespoon fresh lemon juice**
**½ teaspoon dill weed**
**Celery stalks**
**Stuffed green olives, sliced, for garnish**

1. Chop the garlic in a food processor. Add the rest of the ingredients, and process until the mixture is the texture of ricotta cheese.
2. Spread the mixture into washed, cut celery stalks. Garnish with the green olives.

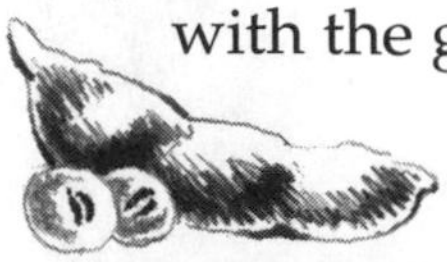

Per 2 tablespoons: Calories 33, Soy Protein 3 g, Total Protein 3 g,
Fat 1 g, Carbohydrates 2 g, Fiber 0 g, Sodium 220 mg

# *Rosemary Oven Fries*

Yield: 4 to 8 servings

*This an easy, savory addition to a quick meal.*

**2 pounds potatoes**
**1 tablespoon oil**
**2 tablespoons red miso**
**1 tablespoon red wine vinegar**
**1 teaspoon garlic powder**
**½ teaspoon rosemary**

1.  Preheat the oven to 400°F.
2. Wash, peel, and slice the potatoes into French-fry shapes.
3. Mix the rest of the ingredients together, pour over the potatoes, and toss until the potato slices are evenly coated.
4. Bake for 20 to 30 minutes until browned, turning once about half way through the cooking.

Per serving: Calories 171, Soy Protein 1 g, Total Protein 3 g,
Fat 2 g, Carbohydrates 34 g, Fiber 3 g, Sodium 348 mg

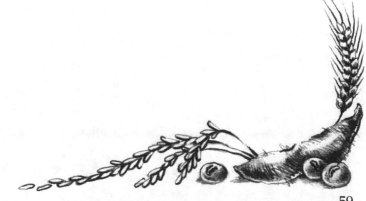

# Snow Peas and Carrots with Tarragon

Yield: 6 servings (about 5 cups)

*This brightly colored vegetable toss will be an appealing warm side dish. You can also chill the vegetables immediately after cooking and serve as a salad.*

**2 cups thinly, diagonally sliced carrots**
**1 pound snow peas**
**1 tablespoon chopped fresh tarragon leaves**
**1 small clove garlic, minced**
**2 tablespoons chick-pea miso**
**1 tablespoon hempseed or extra-virgin olive oil**

1. Boil the carrots for 3 minutes until crisp tender, drain, and put in a bowl.
2. Boil the snow peas for 30 seconds until crisp tender, drain and add to the bowl.
3. Immediately add the rest of the ingredients, toss, and serve.

Per serving: Calories 82, Soy Protein 0 g, Total Protein 3 g,
Fat 2 g, Carbohydrates 11 g, Fiber 5 g, Sodium 316 mg

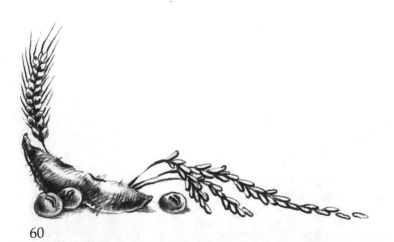

# *Snow Peas with Sesame-Ginger Sauce*

Yield: 2 to 4 servings (2 cups)

*Served as an appetizer, salad, or side dish, these crispy snow peas or green beans will be a welcome treat.*

**½ pound snow peas or baby green beans**
**1 small clove garlic, minced**
**½ teaspoon minced fresh ginger**
**1 tablespoon mellow white miso**
**1 teaspoon sesame oil**
**1 teaspoon sesame seeds**

1. Blanch the snow peas or green beans in boiling water for about 30 seconds, then immediately plunge them into ice water to cool. Drain.

2. Mix the rest of the ingredients with a fork, and toss with the cooled vegetables. Serve cold or reheat, but do not to boil.

Per serving: Calories 66, Soy Protein 1 g, Total Protein 3 g,
Fat 2 g, Carbohydrates 8 g, Fiber 4 g, Sodium 403 mg

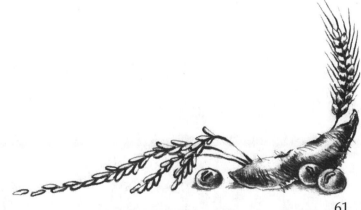

# Spicy Oven Fries

Yield: 4 to 8 servings

*These spicy flavored fries make a tasty accompaniment to almost any meal.*

**2 pounds potatoes**
**2 tablespoons oil**
**3 tablespoons mellow white miso**
**1 tablespoon apple cider vinegar**
**1 teaspoon garlic powder**
**⅛ teaspoon chipotle chile powder, or to taste**

1. Preheat the oven to 400°F.

2. Wash, peel, and slice the potatoes into French fry shapes.

3. Mix the rest of the ingredients together, pour over the potatoes, and toss until the potato slices are evenly coated.

4. Bake for 20 to 25 minutes until browned, turning once about half way through the cooking.

Per serving: Calories 204, Soy Protein 2 g, Total Protein 3 g,
Fat 4 g, Carbohydrates 36 g, Fiber 3 g, Sodium 608 mg

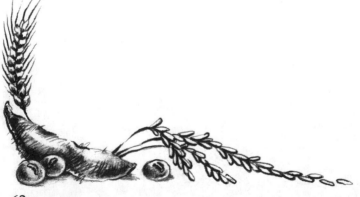

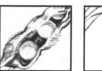

# *Main Dishes*

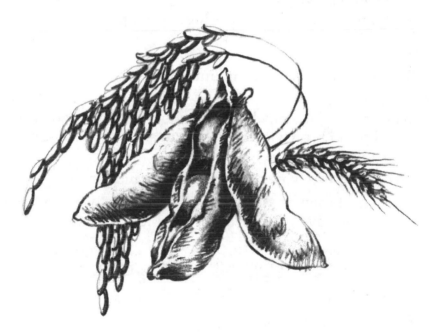

# Marinated Tempeh Sticks

Yield: 2 to 4 servings

*These tasty tempeh sticks can be browned in oil before they are flavored, or they can be marinated and grilled. Browning the sticks first makes them chewier. (They are pictured with the Crispy Crunchy Sweet Pepper Stir-Fry from page 55 on the opposing page and on the cover.)*

**8 ounces tempeh**
**1 tablespoon red or barley miso**
**1 tablespoon balsamic vinegar**
**1 tablespoon water**
**1 small clove garlic**
**1 tablespoon minced fresh ginger (optional)**

First Method:

1. Steam the tempeh for 20 minutes.

2. Cut the steamed tempeh into ¼-inch strips. In a nonstick pan, brown the tempeh on one side in ½ tablespoon of olive oil. Flip and brown the other side in another ½ tablespoon of olive oil. Turn off the heat.

3. Blend the miso, vinegar, water, garlic, and ginger.

4. While the browned sticks are still hot, pour the miso mixture over them, cover, and let stand for a few minutes.

Per serving: Calories 201, Soy Protein 13 g, Total Protein 13 g,
Fat 8 g, Carbohydrates 14 g, Fiber 4 g, Sodium 345 mg

Second Method:

1. Steam the tempeh for 20 minutes.

2. Blend the miso, vinegar, water, garlic, and ginger.

3. Cut the steamed tempeh into ¼-inch strips, arrange in a glass or stainless pan, and pour the miso mixture evenly over the strips. Marinate for a few hours or overnight.

4. Brown on a hot grill.

Per serving: Calories 161, Soy Protein 13 g, Total Protein 13 g,
Fat 5 g, Carbohydrates 14 g, Fiber 4 g, Sodium 345 mg

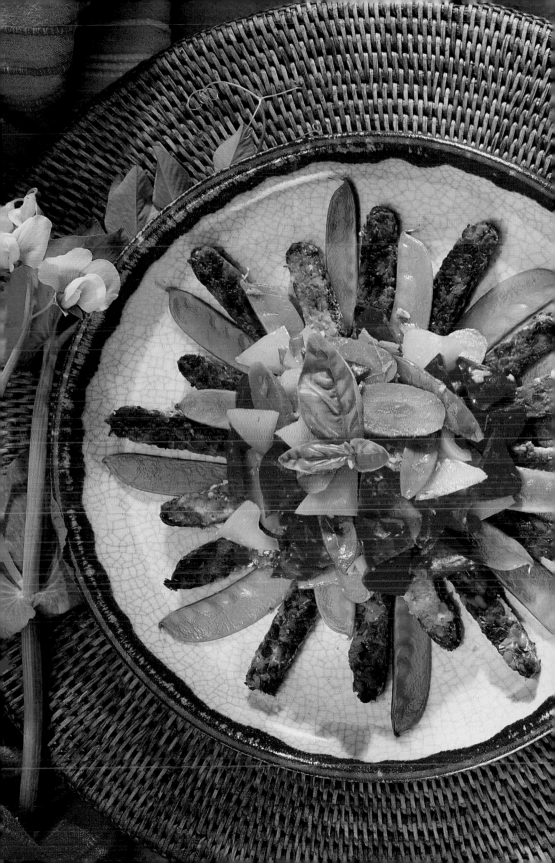

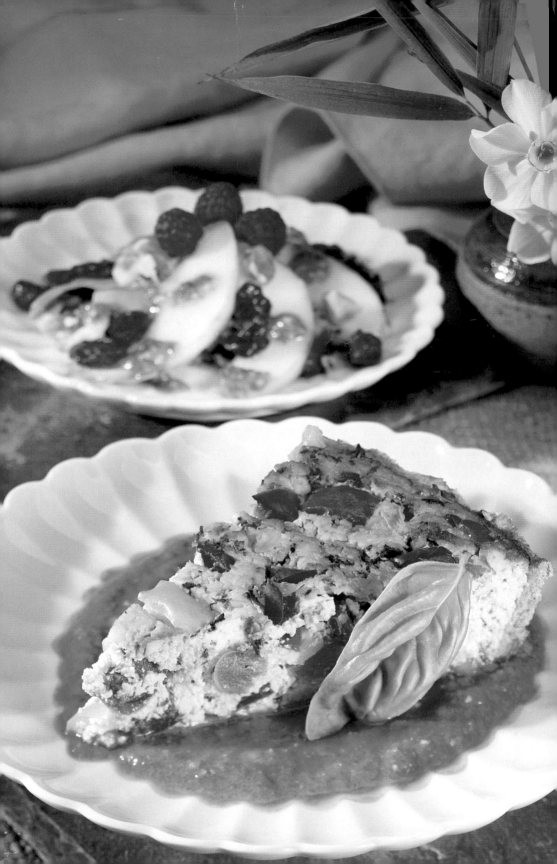

# Sweet Pepper Onion Quiche

Yield: 1 (9-inch) quiche (6 to 8 servings)

*This colorful quiche is pictured with Roasted Red Pepper Dip (page 21) on the opposing page.*

**Your favorite crust (optional)**
**2 cups chopped red, yellow, and green bell peppers**
**2 cups chopped onions**
**2 cloves garlic, minced**
**2 tablespoons olive oil**
**2 pounds tofu**
**¼ cup sweet white miso**
**¼ cup nutritional yeast**
**3 tablespoons chopped fresh parsley (¼ ounce)**
**3 tablespoons chopped fresh basil (¼ ounce)**

1. Preheat the oven to 350°F. If you are using a crust, prebake it for about 10 minutes.

2. Sauté the peppers, onions, and garlic in the olive oil.

3. Blend the tofu, miso, and nutritional yeast in a food processor. Combine all the ingredients in a bowl, mix well, and pour into a quiche pan, with or without the pre-baked crust.

4. Bake for about 1 hour, or until the top starts to brown and form cracks. Let cool a few minutes before serving.

Per serving: Calories 195, Soy Protein 11 g, Total Protein 13 g,
Fat 1 g, Carbohydrates 11 g, Fiber 2 g, Sodium 515 mg

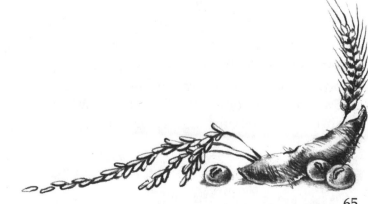

# Crepes

Yield: 4 to 5 (10-inch) crepes

*Serve these crepes filled with steamed vegetables or sliced, sautéed porto-bello mushrooms and topped with Miso Gravy (page 52).*

**½ cup unbleached flour**
**1 cup unflavored soymilk**
**1 tablespoon sweet miso, or ½ tablespoon red miso**
**1 tablespoon nutritional yeast (optional)**
**¼ teaspoon baking powder**

1. Combine all the ingredients in a blender until smooth.

2. Pour about ⅓ cup of the batter into a hot 10-inch, oiled crepe pan, tilting and turning the pan until the batter evenly covers the bottom. Turn the crepe when it starts to pull away from the edge of the pan and is browned underneath. Let the other side brown, and remove from the pan.

Per crepe: Calories 72, Soy Protein 2 g, Total Protein 3 g,
Fat 1 g, Carbohydrates 12 g, Fiber 1 g, Sodium 200 mg

# Jerk Tofu

Yield: 3 to 4 servings

*Here is a taste of the Caribbean with a tofu base.*

**1 pound tofu, frozen, thawed, and squeezed dry**
**1 cup Jerk Sauce (page 45)**

1. Preheat the oven to 350°F.

2. Cut the tofu into ¼-inch slices, then into ½-inch bite-sized pieces, and place in a bowl.

3. Pour the Miso-Jerk Sauce over the tofu. Using rubber gloves, press the sauce into the tofu pieces.

4. Spread the pieces out on an oiled baking sheet, and bake for 15 minutes on one side. Flip them over and bake about 10 more minutes until lightly browned.

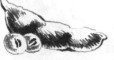

Per serving: Calories 88, Soy Protein 5 g, Total Protein 5 g,
Fat 2 g, Carbohydrates 11 g, Fiber 0 g, Sodium 260 mg

# Tofu Nuggets

Yield: 3 to 4 servings

*This is a quick and easy chewy tofu dish.*

**1 pound tofu, frozen, thawed, and squeezed dry**
**2 cloves garlic**
**1 ounce onion (a good sized slice)**
**2 tablespoons mellow barley miso**
**2 tablespoons unsalted cashew butter**
**¼ cup water**

1. Preheat the oven to 350°F.
2. Cut the tofu into ¾-inch cubes, and set them aside in a bowl.
3. Combine the garlic and onion in a blender until chopped.
4. Add the miso, cashew butter, and water, and blend until creamy.
5. Pour the mixture over the tofu cubes, and press it into the cubes until it is all absorbed or coating the outside.
6. Arrange the cubes on an oiled baking sheet, and bake for 10 minutes. Turn the cubes and bake on the opposite side until browned, about 10 minutes more.

Per serving: Calories 181, Soy Protein 11 g, Total Protein 12 g,
Fat 10 g, Carbohydrates 8 g, Fiber 1 g, Sodium 508 mg

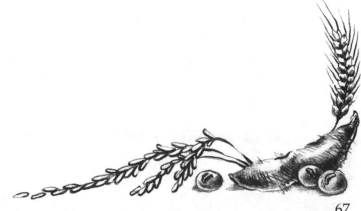

# Marinated Tofu

Yield: 2 servings

*Here are six different marinades for tofu using different types of miso. Each recipe is enough for ½ pound of tofu. They can be used with either fresh regular tofu or frozen tofu that has been thawed and carefully squeezed dry. Eliminate the water in the recipes if you use regular tofu. Cut the tofu into ¼- x ½- x 1-inch pieces or ½-inch cubes. Mix the marinade, pour over the tofu, and marinate overnight or at least for a few hours. You can brown the tofu in a pan with olive oil or bake it on an oiled baking sheet at 350°F for 20 minutes, turning the pieces once halfway through.*

### Red Miso Ginger Marinade

**1 to 2 tablespoons red miso**
**2 tablespoons water**
**1 tablespoon balsamic vinegar**
**2 teaspoons minced fresh ginger**
**1 small clove garlic, minced**

> Per serving: Calories 16, Soy Protein 2 g, Total Protein 2 g, Fat 0 g, Carbohydrates 2 g, Fiber 0 g, Sodium 510 mg

### Sweet White Tahini Marinade

**2 to 3 tablespoons sweet white miso, or**
    **2 tablespoons sweet barley miso**
**2 tablespoons rice vinegar**
**1 tablespoon water**
**1 tablespoon mirin**
**1 tablespoon unsalted tahini**
**1 small clove garlic, minced**

> Per serving: Calories 145, Soy Protein 4 g, Total Protein 3 g, Fat 2 g, Carbohydrates 18 g, Fiber 1 g, Sodium 1011 mg

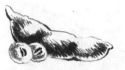

### Roasted Almond-Miso Marinade

**1 to 2 tablespoons brown rice miso**
**2 tablespoons wine vinegar**
**2 tablespoons water**
**1 tablespoon unsalted almond butter**
**1 teaspoon basil**
**1 clove garlic minced**

> Per serving: Calories 68, Soy Protein 2 g, Total Protein 3 g,
> Fat 4 g, Carbohydrates 4 g, Fiber 0 g, Sodium 511 mg

### Middle Eastern Marinade

**2 to 3 tablespoons sweet white or chick-pea miso**
**2 tablespoons lemon juice**
**2 tablespoons water**
**1 tablespoon tahini**
**1 small clove garlic, minced**
**½ teaspoon dill weed**

> Per serving: Calories 62, Soy Protein 5 g, Total Protein 2 g,
> Fat 2 g, Carbohydrates 5 g, Fiber 1 g, Sodium 296 mg

### Mellow Barley and Lemon Basil Marinade

**1 to 2 tablespoons mellow barley miso**
**1 tablespoon lemon juice**
**2 tablespoons water**
**½ teaspoon basil**
**1 clove garlic, minced**

> Per serving: Calories 25, Soy Protein 2 g, Total Protein 2 g,
> Fat 0 g, Carbohydrates 3 g, Fiber 0 g, Sodium 435 mg

### Mellow White Ginger Marinade

**1 to 2 tablespoons mellow white miso**
**2 tablespoons mirin**
**1 tablespoon water**
**2 tablespoons sweetener of choice**
**2 teaspoons minced fresh ginger**
**1 small clove garlic, minced**

> Per serving: Calories 193, Soy Protein 2 g, Total Protein 2 g,
> Fat 0 g, Carbohydrates 40 g, Fiber 0 g, Sodium 871 mg

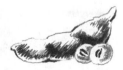

# Mushroom-Onion Quiche

Yield: 1 (9-inch) quiche (6 to 8 servings)

*Try this for a brunch, luncheon, or casual dinner.*

**Your favorite crust (optional)**
**1 pound mushrooms**
**1 cup chopped onions**
**2 cloves garlic, minced**
**1 tablespoon olive oil**
**2 pounds tofu**
**3 tablespoons red miso**

1. Preheat the oven to 350°F. If you are using a crust, prebake it for about 10 minutes.

2. Sauté the mushrooms, onions, and garlic in the olive oil.

3. Blend tofu and miso together in a food processor. Mix all the ingredients and pour into a quiche pan, with or without the pre-baked crust.

4. Bake for about 1 hour, or until the top starts to brown and form cracks. Let cool a few minutes before serving.

Per serving: Calories 154, Soy Protein 10 g, Total Protein 11 g,
Fat 7 g, Carbohydrates 8 g, Fiber 2 g, Sodium 451 mg

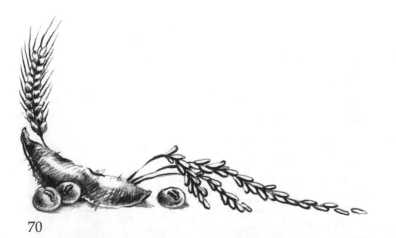

# Split Mung Dahl

Yield: 6 to 8 servings

*This is a simple and tasty meal that always pleases. If you cannot find split mung dahl, substitute yellow split peas or any other dahl you like.*

**2 cups split mung dahl (1 pound)**
**6 cups boiling water**
**3 onions, sliced**
**¼ cup oil**
**3 tablespoons curry powder, or to taste**
**¼ cup apple cider vinegar, or to taste**
**¼ cup red miso**
**1 cup hot water**

1. Wash and sort the mung dahl, add to the boiling water, and simmer until soft, about 30 minutes.

2. Sauté the onions in the oil until transparent. Stir in the curry powder, and continue to cook over low heat for a few minutes until the curry powder has a toasted aroma.

3. Stir the onion-curry mixture into the soft mung dahl along with the vinegar, and turn off the heat.

4. Dissolve the miso in the hot water, and stir into the dahl. Serve over basmati rice with soy yogurt and your favorite chutney.

Per serving: Calories 187, Soy Protein 2 g, Total Protein 7 g,
Fat 8 g, Carbohydrates 21 g, Fiber 4 g, Sodium 586 mg

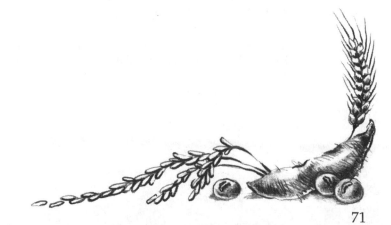

# Taco or Burrito Filling

Yield: 2½ cups

*This makes a chewy, tasty filling for tacos, burritos, enchiladas, and more.*

**⅞ cup boiling water or tomato juice**
**¼ cup salsa of choice**
**1 cup textured soy protein granules**
**½ cup finely chopped onions**
**½ cup finely chopped green bell peppers**
**Jalapeño or other hot pepper, chopped (use to taste)**
**1 clove garlic, minced**
**1 tablespoon olive oil**
**1 tablespoon chili powder**
**2 tablespoons red miso**
**½ cup hot water**

1. Mix the boiling water and salsa, and pour over the soy protein granules; let stand for about 10 minutes.
2. Sauté the onions, green peppers, jalapeño, and garlic in the olive oil until the onions are transparent. Stir in the chili powder, and let simmer for a few minutes.
3. Mix in the soy protein granules, and continue cooking until they start to brown.
4. Dissolve the miso in the hot water, and pour it over the vegetable-soy mixture; stir and turn off the heat. Cover and let stand until all the liquid is absorbed.

Per ¼ cup: Calories 50, Soy Protein 5 g, Total Protein 5 g,
Fat 1 g, Carbohydrates 4 g, Fiber 1 g, Sodium 226 mg

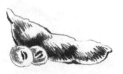

# *Tempeh Pâté*

Yield: about 2½ cups

*Here are two differently flavored pâtés to spread on crackers or bread.*

### Red Miso Pâté

8 ounces tempeh
1 large onion, chopped
4 cloves garlic, minced
1 tablespoon olive oil
1 ounce fresh parsley
1 teaspoon thyme
3 tablespoons red miso

### Barley Miso Pâté

8 ounces tempeh
1 large onion, chopped
4 cloves garlic, minced
1 tablespoon olive oil
1 ounce fresh parsley
1 teaspoon savory
4 tablespoons barley miso

1. Steam the tempeh for 20 minutes, and set aside to cool.
2. Sauté the onion and garlic in the olive oil until the onion is caramelized.
3. In a food processor, chop the onion and garlic and parsley. Add the rest of ingredients and blend until smooth.

Per 2 tablespoons (Red Miso): Calories 36, Soy Protein 2 g, Total Protein 2 g, Fat 2 g, Carbohydrates 3 g, Fiber 1 g, Sodium 154 mg

Per 2 tablespoons (Barley Miso): Calories 41, Soy Protein 2 g, Total Protein 3 g, Fat 2 g, Carbohydrates 4 g, Fiber 1 g, Sodium 127 mg

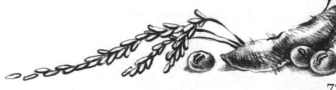

# Holiday Vital Wheat Gluten Roast

Yield: 6 servings

*This is a substantial, festive holiday entrée, surrounded with a savory gravy, and with no added fat. You can prepare this ahead of time, and freeze at the point it is ready to go in to the oven. Thaw before baking. (Pictured on the back cover.)*

1 tablespoon unsalted almond butter
2 tablespoons red miso or other dark miso
1 tablespoon onion powder
1 teaspoon garlic powder
¼ teaspoon freshly ground black pepper
½ teaspoon sage
½ teaspoon thyme
2 tablespoons dry red wine (optional)
1 cup room temperature water
1 cup vital wheat gluten

1½ cups hot water
2 tablespoons red miso or other dark miso
2 tablespoons dry red wine (optional)

1 carrot, cut in half
1 rib celery, cut in half
1 large clove garlic
1 small onion, quartered

1 tablespoon unbleached flour

1. In a blender, combine the almond butter, 2 tablespoons miso, onion powder, garlic powder, black pepper, sage, thyme, 2 tablespoons wine, and 1 cup water.

2. Pour the mixture into the vital wheat gluten, and gently mix. Form into an even thickness to fit your steamer basket. Place it in the steamer basket of a 6-quart pressure cooker.

3. Mix the 1½ cups hot water, 2 tablespoons miso, and 2 tablespoons wine, and pour over the gluten.

4. Place the carrot, celery, garlic, and onion on top of the roast.

5. Pressure cook at 15 pounds for 1 hour. Remove the roast and cut into ⅛- to ¼-inch slices. Arrange in a baking dish or roasting pan.

6. In a blender, combine the cooking liquid and vegetables with the 1 tablespoon flour, and pour over the slices in the roasting pan. Cover and bake at 350°F for about 30 minutes. Serve along with baked potatoes, sweet potatoes, and/or winter squash.

Per serving: Calories 134, Soy Protein 2 g, Total Protein 21 g,
Fat 2 g, Carbohydrates 7 g, Fiber 1 g, Sodium 690 mg

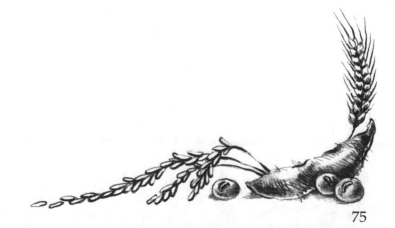

# Thai Green Curry

Yield: 4 servings

*Make this one as hot as you like. It takes a bit of preparation, but is well worth the effort. The vegan version of green curry paste is the base of this recipe. Curry paste usually involves fish or shrimp paste, but the miso more than makes up for the fish flavor.*

### Green Curry Sauce

- 1 teaspoon black peppercorns
- 1 teaspoon cumin seeds
- 2 teaspoons coriander seeds
- 4 large Thai chilis or one Anaheim chili, without stems and seeds, chopped (add to taste)
- 2 teaspoons minced fresh ginger (¼ ounce)
- 1 medium sweet onion, chopped
- 2 large cloves garlic, minced
- ½ cup chopped fresh cilantro
- ½ cup chopped fresh basil
- 2 teaspoons lemon or lime zest
- 2 teaspoons turmeric
- 1 tablespoon canola oil
- 1 (13.5-ounce) can coconut milk
- ½ cup water

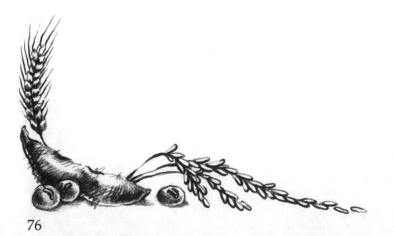

½ pound tofu, frozen, thawed, squeezed dry,
and torn into bite-sized pieces
½ pound green beans or sugar snap peas
1 teaspoon canola oil
½ pound red bell pepper, cut into 1-inch chunks
¼ cup chopped basil
¼ cup chopped cilantro
2 tablespoons red miso, or 4 tablespoons
mellow white miso
½ cup hot water

1. Toast the peppercorns, cumin seeds, and coriander seeds in a
   hot dry pan for 1 to 3 minutes until their aroma is apparent.
   Grind in a spice or coffee grinder.

2. In a food processor combine the chilis, ginger, onion, garlic,
   ½ cup cilantro, ½ cup basil, and lime zest until puréed. Add
   the turmeric and ground spice mixture, and blend.

3. Cook for about 2 minutes over medium heat in the 1 tablespoon canola oil, or until the aroma becomes strong. Stir in
   the coconut milk and water, and simmer.

4. Sauté the tofu and red pepper in the 1 teaspoon canola oil
   until the tofu is slightly browned. Add the tofu/red pepper
   mixture, green beans, ¼ cup basil, and ¼ cup cilantro to the
   simmering sauce. Continue cooking for about 5 minutes, or
   until the vegetables are crisp tender.

5. Dissolve the miso in the hot water, turn off the heat
   under the saucepan, and stir in the miso. Press on the
   tofu pieces, so they will soak up the sauce. Serve over
   rice.

Per serving: Calories 374, Soy Protein 5 g, Total Protein 9 g,
Fat 25 g, Carbohydrates 15 g, Fiber 5 g, Sodium 534 mg

# Tofu Ribs

Yield: 6 servings

*These chewy, spicy "ribs" sit well between buns for a sandwich. Try serving with Spicy Oven Fries (page 62).*

**1½ pounds tofu, frozen, thawed, and squeezed dry**
**1 clove garlic**
**1 to 2 tablespoons brown rice miso**
**2 tablespoons unsalted nut butter**
**¼ cup water**
**1 recipe Old Time Barbecue Sauce (page 43)**

1. Preheat the oven to 350°F.

2. Cut the tofu into ½- x ½-inch strips.

3. In a small blender or food processor, chop the garlic, then add the miso, nut butter, and water, and blend until smooth.

4. In a shallow pan, pour the mixture over the tofu strips, and press it in.

5. Spread out the tofu strips on an oiled baking sheet. Bake for 15 minutes on one side, flip over, and bake for 5 minutes on the other side. Pour the barbecue sauce over all, and bake for 5 more minutes.

Per serving: Calories 251, Soy Protein 10 g, Total Protein 13 g,
Fat 9 g, Carbohydrates 25 g, Fiber 2 g, Sodium 813 mg

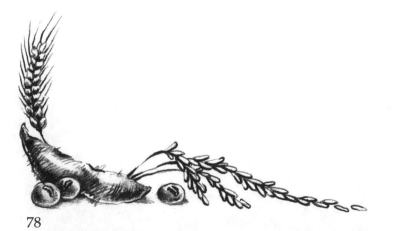

# *Side Dishes*

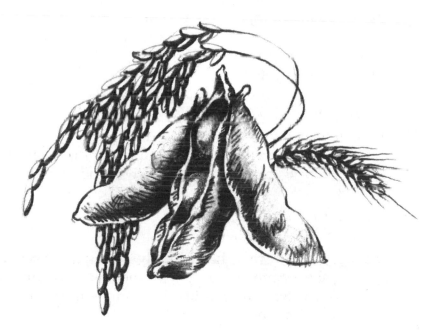

# Miso Garlic Bread

Yield: 1 loaf Italian Bread (12 slices)

*Any flavor of miso can be used for this unique, cheesy-tasting, crunchy garlic bread treat. Try using rye or whole grain bread or a different miso on each half of the loaf for variety in a meal. Time this one to come out of the oven at the very last minute before sitting down at the table.*

**10 cloves garlic**
**6 tablespoons olive oil**
**3 tablespoons light miso (such as sweet white**
**or chick-pea), or 2 tablespoons dark miso**
**(such as red or barley)**
**2 tablespoons chopped fresh basil**
**or minced chives, or 1 teaspoon**
**dried basil (optional)**
**1 loaf Italian bread**

1. Preheat the oven to 500°F.

2. Toast the unpeeled garlic cloves in a dry skillet, tossing over medium high heat for about 8 minutes, until they are fragrant and starting to change color; cool and remove the skins.

3. Mash the garlic in a bowl, and whip together with the olive oil and miso. Mix in the herbs.

4. Cut the bread lengthways, horizontally, laying it cut side up on a baking sheet. Spread evenly with the miso mixture, and bake for 5 to 8 minutes until crispy and golden. Cut into slices and serve hot.

Per slice: Calories 156, Soy Protein 1 g, Total Protein 4 g,
Fat 7 g, Carbohydrates 18 g, Fiber 1 g, Sodium 394 mg

# Mushroom Sauté

Yield: about 2 cups

*Serve this savory mushroom blend as a wrap or on grilled French bread, for an appetizer, or as part of a meal. (See these served as bruchettas in the picture opposite page 33.)*

½ pound fresh mushrooms (shiitake or other special
　variety), sliced
1 medium onion, chopped
2 cloves garlic, minced
1 tablespoon olive oil
½ cup chopped fresh parsley
¼ teaspoon thyme
¼ teaspoon marjoram
1 tablespoon barley or red miso
¼ cup hot water

1. Sauté the mushrooms, onion, and garlic in the olive oil. When the onions are soft, stir in the parsley, thyme, and marjoram, and continue to cook over low heat.
2. Dissolve the miso in the hot water.
3. Turn off the heat under the mushrooms. Pour the miso over the mushrooms, stir, and simmer for a few minutes until the liquid evaporates.

Per ¼ cup: Calories 34, Soy Protein 1 g, Total Protein 1 g,
Fat 1 g, Carbohydrates 3 g, Fiber 1 g, Sodium 131 mg

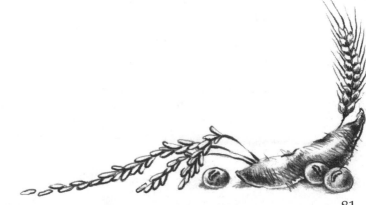

# *Risotto Delicata*

Yield: 4 to 6 servings

*This savory and mildly sweet mix could be a main dish or a side dish.*

> **1 pound delicata squash**
> **1 tablespoon olive oil**
> **1 large leek or onion, chopped (about 1½ cups), light parts only**
> **1 clove garlic, minced**
> **1 tablespoon olive oil**
> **1 cup medium grain white rice**
> **3 cups boiling water**
> **½ (12.3-ounce package) silken tofu**
> **1 tablespoon red miso**

1. Preheat the oven to 350°F.
2. Cut the squash in half and remove the seeds. Cut it into ¾-inch cubes.
3. Toss the squash cubes with 1 tablespoon olive oil, and spread on an oiled baking sheet. Cover and bake until the squash is tender and begins to caramelize, about 40 minutes.
4. Sauté the leek and garlic in 1 tablespoon olive oil until transparent.
5. Add the rice to the leeks, and stir until the rice is coated and slightly toasted.
6. Add the boiling water ½ cup at a time. Simmer and stir until the liquid is absorbed.
7. Blend the tofu and miso together. Stir into the rice along with the squash cubes. Serve hot.

Per serving: Calories 223, Soy Protein 3 g, Total Protein 6 g,
Fat 7 g, Carbohydrates 34 g, Fiber 3 g, Sodium 225 mg

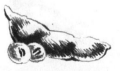

# Soba and Spinach Toss

Yield: 6 to 8 servings

**12 ounces soba (buckwheat noodles)**
**1 onion, chopped**
**1 small medium hot red pepper, chopped**
**1 green bell pepper, chopped**
**2 cloves garlic, minced**
**1 tablespoon olive oil**
**1 large bag frozen spinach, or 2 bunches fresh spinach,**
  **washed**

*Sauce*
**2 tablespoons olive oil**
**1 tablespoon sweet white miso**
**1 tablespoon chick-pea miso**
**1 clove garlic, minced**
**2 teaspoons minced fresh ginger (¼ ounce)**
**1 teaspoon orange zest**

1. Cook the soba according to package directions, and drain.
2. Sauté the onion, peppers, and 2 cloves of the minced garlic in 1 tablespoon of olive oil until the onions are transparent.
3. Add the spinach, cover, and cook over medium heat until the spinach either thaws, if using frozen, or wilts if using fresh.
4. Blend together the 2 tablespoons of olive oil, with the miso, 1 clove minced garlic, ginger, and orange zest.
5. Toss all together and serve hot.

Per serving: Calories 258, Soy Protein 0 g, Total Protein 7 g,
Fat 6 g, Carbohydrates 41 g, Fiber 2 g, Sodium 291 mg

# Spinach and Tofu

Yield: 2½ cups

*Serve this as a side dish, a light main dish or as a filling in turnovers or pie.*

**1 medium onion, chopped**
**1 clove garlic, minced**
**1 tablespoon olive oil**
**½ pound tofu, cubed or crumbled**
**½ pound spinach, chopped**
**1½ tablespoons mellow white miso**
**¼ cup hot water**

1. Sauté the onion and garlic in the olive oil until they caramelize.
2. Add the tofu and spinach, cover, and cook over low heat until the spinach shrinks and softens, about 5 minutes.
3. Dissolve the miso in the hot water, pour over the mixture in the pan, and gently stir. Turn off the heat, cover, and let steep for a few minutes before serving.

Per ½ cup: Calories 92, Soy Protein 4 g, Total Protein 5 g,
Fat 4 g, Carbohydrates 6 g, Fiber 2 g, Sodium 400 mg

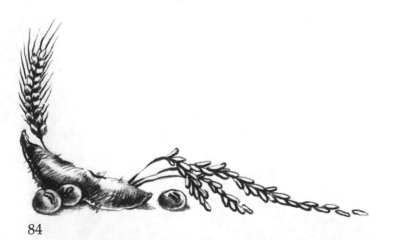

# *Chick-Pea Flour Crepes*

Yield: 4 (8-inch) crepes

*Chick-pea flour and miso are the protein base for these savory crepes. Fill them with sautéed vegetables or Marinated Tempeh (page 64) and top with Miso Gravy (page 52). These crepes are delicate, so handle with care.*

**¾ cup chick-pea flour**
**1 tablespoon mellow barley miso**
**Enough water to make 1½ cups**

1. Combine all the ingredients in a blender until smooth. Add enough water to make a total volume of 1½ cups. Blend until smooth. Let the batter rest for about 30 minutes.

2. Oil and heat a 12-inch, nonstick crepe pan that can be put under the broiler. Turn the broiler to medium-high heat.

3. Blend the batter once, and pour about ½ cup into the pan, turning and tilting the pan to evenly cover the bottom with the batter. When the crepe looks set, after about 4 minutes, place it under the broiler until browned. Stack the finished crepes in towel to keep them warm.

Per crepe: Calories 86, Soy Protein 1 g, Total Protein 5 g,
Fat 1 g, Carbohydrates 14 g, Fiber 3 g, Sodium 221 mg

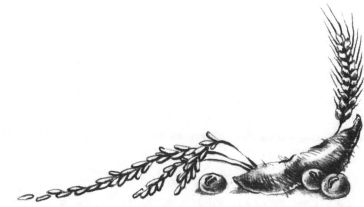

# Couscous, Tofu, and Peas

Yield: 5 cups

*Quick and easy, this can be a side dish or a light main dish.*

**1 clove garlic, minced**
**1 small onion, chopped**
**1 tablespoon olive oil**
**½ teaspoon cumin**
**1½ cups water**
**1 cup frozen peas**
**½ pound firm tofu, cut into small cubes**
**¼ cup sweet white miso, or 3 tablespoons red miso**
**1 cup couscous**

1. Sauté the onion and garlic in the olive oil until transparent. Add the cumin and continue to cook for about 1 minute.

2. In a saucepan, bring the water to a boil, add the frozen peas and tofu, return to a boil, and cook for 1 minute. Turn off the heat.

3. Dissolve the miso into the hot liquid, stir in the onion mixture and couscous, cover, and let stand for about 5 minutes. Fluff with a fork and serve.

Per cup: Calories 220, Soy Protein 6 g, Total Protein 10 g,
Fat 4 g, Carbohydrates 31 g, Fiber 5 g, Sodium 704 mg

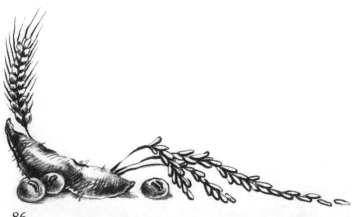

# *Asparagus and Pasta Toss*

Yield: 4 servings (5 cups)

*This is an asparagus treat not to be missed.*

**½ pound bow tie pasta**
**2 cloves garlic, minced**
**1 small onion, sliced**
**2 tablespoons olive oil**
**1 pound asparagus, trimmed and cut into 2-inch pieces**
**¼ cup water**
**2 tablespoons mellow white miso**
**1 tablespoon wine vinegar**

1. Cook the pasta in boiling water for about 12 minutes, or until al dente, and drain.
2. While the pasta is cooking, sauté the garlic and onion in 1 tablespoon of the olive oil. Add the asparagus, toss, add the water, cover, and steam for 7 minutes.
3. Blend together the remaining 1 tablespoon olive oil, miso, and vinegar.
4. When the asparagus is tender, turn off the heat and mix in the miso mixture. Toss all together with the pasta, and serve.

Per serving: Calories 180, Soy Protein 2 g, Total Protein 6 g,
Fat 77 g, Carbohydrates 22 g, Fiber 3 g, Sodium 606 mg

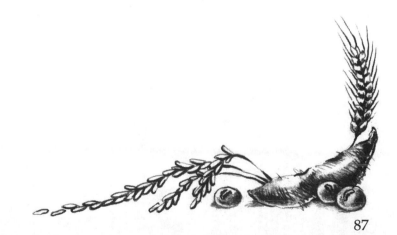

# Soba and Sesame Sauce

Yield: 2 servings

*Here is a quick and easy side dish that can accompany many different dishes.*

**1 clove garlic, minced**
**1 tablespoon mellow white miso**
**1 tablespoon sesame oil**
**½ tablespoon sesame seeds**
**Pinch of cayenne (optional)**
**¼ pound soba (buckwheat noodles),**
    **cooked and drained**

1. Blend the garlic, miso, sesame oil, sesame seeds, and cayenne together with a small blender, small wire whip, or fork.
2. Toss with the hot soba, and serve.

Per serving: Calories 299, Soy Protein 2 g, Total Protein 8 g,
Fat 8 g, Carbohydrates 46 g, Fiber 0 g, Sodium 600 mg

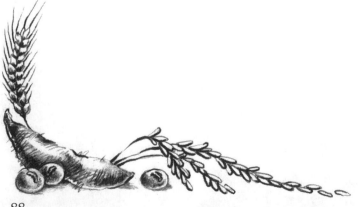

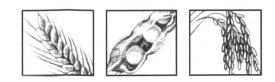

# *Sweet Things*

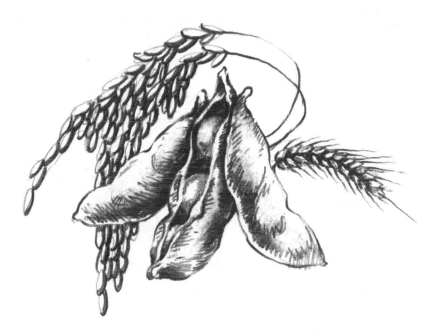

# Gingerbread

Yield: 1 round (8-inch) cake (8 servings)

*Two different kinds of ginger and some red miso spice up this ginger-bread.*

**¼ cup oil**
**1 cup sorghum or molasses**
**¼ cup minced fresh ginger**
**2 teaspoons powdered ginger**
**2 tablespoons red miso**
**2 cups unbleached or whole wheat flour**
**1 teaspoon baking soda**
**1 cup hot water**

1. Preheat the oven to 350°F.
2. Beat together the oil, sorghum, fresh ginger, powdered ginger, and miso.
3. Beat in the flour and baking soda.
4. Beat in the hot water, and pour into an 8-inch round pan. Bake for 30 to 40 minutes.

Per serving: Calories 308, Soy Protein 1 g, Total Protein 4 g,
Fat 7 g, Carbohydrates 57 g, Fiber 1 g, Sodium 311 mg

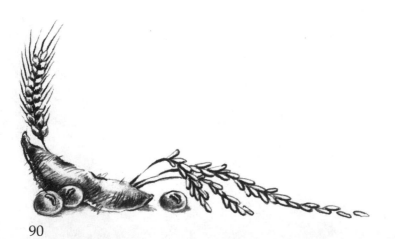

# Baked Stuffed Pears with Sauce

Yield: 4 to 8 servings

*Here is a new version of an old-time recipe. The sweet miso complements the fruit and brings out the flavors.*

**4 pears or apples**
**1 tablespoon sweet white, sweet barley,**
**    or chick-pea miso**
**½ cup hot water**
**3 tablespoons chopped dried fruit**
**    (figs, apricots, etc.)**
**½ teaspoon cinnamon**
**1 tablespoon fresh lemon juice**
**1 tablespoon chopped candied ginger**
**3 tablespoons chopped nuts (walnuts, pecans,**
**    almonds, etc.)**

1. Cut the pears or apples in half, and scoop out the core with a rounded tablespoon or melon baller.
2. Dissolve the miso in the hot water, add the dried fruit, and let stand until softened.
3. Stir in the cinnamon, lemon juice, candied ginger, and nuts.
4. Preheat the oven to 350°F.
5. Arrange the fruit in a baking pan, with the scooped side up and fill with the filling. Pour enough water in the pan to cover the bottom. Cover and bake until the fruit is soft, about 20 to 25 minutes.

Per serving: Calories 145, Soy Protein 1 g, Total Protein 2 g, Fat 3 g, Carbohydrates 28 g, Fiber 5 g, Sodium 148 mg

# *Peach Soy Frogurt*

Yield: about 5 cups

*Sweet miso blends well with fruit. Start this frogurt mix with frozen peaches and you won't have to chill the mix before pouring it into the ice cream machine. If you can't find it already made, soy yogurt can be made with plain soymilk and an active yogurt starter.*

**1 pound frozen or fresh peach slices (3cups)**
**2 cups soy yogurt**
**½ cup sweetener of choice**
**1 tablespoon sweet white miso**
**1 teaspoon vanilla extract**

1. Blend all the ingredients together until smooth. If you are using fresh peaches, chill the mixture at least 4 hours, or until thoroughly chilled.

2. Pour into an ice cream machine and run it for about 20 minutes until frozen. Serve immediately or store in the freezer.

Per serving: Calories 184, Soy Protein 3 g, Total Protein 3 g,
Fat 1 g, Carbohydrates 38 g, Fiber 3 g, Sodium 188 mg

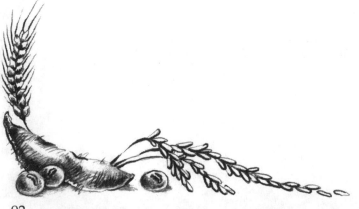

# *Fruit and Nut Pie*

Yield: 1 (nine-inch) pie (8 to 10 servings)

*This is a unique sweet-salty fruit pie much like the holiday treat mincemeat. The dark miso compliments the sweet tartness of the fruit.*

**2 cups chopped mixed dried fruit**
**1¼ cups orange juice or mixed fruit juice**
**2 Granny Smith or other tart apples, chopped**
   **(about 4 cups)**
**1 tablespoon organic orange zest**
**1 cup chopped walnuts**
**1 tablespoon cornstarch**
**½ teaspoon cinnamon**
**¼ teaspoon allspice**
**¼ teaspoon nutmeg**
**¼ cup apple juice**
**1 tablespoon red or barley miso**

**1 baked 9-inch pie shell**

1. In a saucepan, combine all the ingredients, except the apple juice and miso, and bring to a boil. Reduce the heat to a simmer, and cook until the apples are almost soft.

2. Mix the apple juice and miso, turn off the heat under the fruit mixture, and stir in the miso mixture.

3. Pour the mixture into the baked pie shell, and cool before serving.

Per serving: Calories 333, Soy Protein 0 g, Total Protein 4 g,
Fat 14 g, Carbohydrates 46 g, Fiber 5 g, Sodium 247 mg

# Index

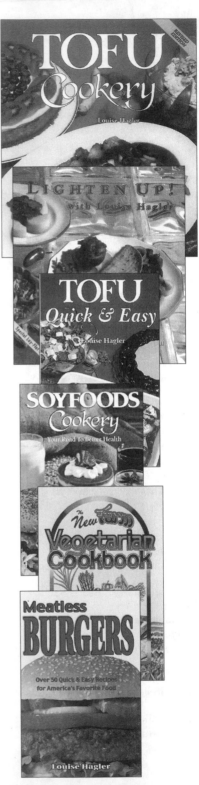